INTRODUCTION

This book is a selection of information that I have found to be very helpful over the last two years. As I researched for information on different topics I thought it would be nice to put all my findings in a book that may be helpful to others. Some of these remedies I have tried and they work and I still use them today.

My life has changed because of many herbs and vitamins and I hope this book will help you in the same way.

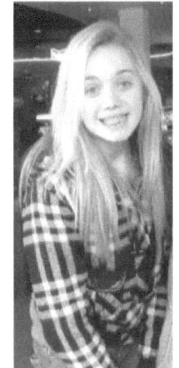

Join me as I fill you in on all the information that I have learned. This book is about Vitamins, Minerals, Healthy Eating, lots of Sleep and Exercise. I have also included some great tips on making your own lotions, makeup and other items I am sure you will enjoy.

Go get yourself a green tea, light a candle, relax and read.

Let's start with Vitamins.. Many of us lack many vitamins as we do not eat a healthy diet. Some of us are too busy and don't stop and think about our health until it is too late and we are sick. Then we go to the drugstore and buy all these medications to help get rid of our ailments.. There are many tips in here that will help you live a healthier life just by taking a little time to understand our body and what we need to do to stay healthy.

CONTENTS

- Vitamins – Page 3
- Herbs for Healing – Page 24
- A Few Great Tips – Page 65
- Hydrogen Peroxide – Page 77
- Benefits of Chocolate – Page 88
- Olive Oil & Coconut Oil – Page 95

VITAMINS

First let's read about Vitamins, many think that just children need Vitamins because they are growing but that is not true, we all may need Vitamins. For many years I thought I ate a fairly good diet and that I was healthy but after reading up on Vitamins and Health issues I realized that I was in need of some good Vitamins. Here is a list of the Vitamins and what they can do to help your body.

Vitamins are a group of substances that are essential for normal cell function, growth, and development.

Before making any changes to your diet or adding vitamin supplements, consult with your physician and have your blood levels tested to check for any deficiencies. If you are taking any medication, make sure you physician is aware of these as some medications can affect the body's ability to absorb vitamins and nutrients, so you may need extra supplementation.

There are 13 essential vitamins, meaning they are needed for the body to function.

Vitamin A

Vitamin C

Vitamin D

Vitamin E

Vitamin K

Vitamin B1 (thiamine)

Vitamin B2 (riboflavin)

Vitamin B3 (niacin)

Pantothenic acid

Biotin

Vitamin B6

Vitamin B12

Folate (folic acid)

Vitamins are grouped into two categories:

Fat-soluble vitamins are stored in the body's fatty tissue. The four fat-soluble vitamins are vitamins A, D, E, and K.

There are nine water-soluble vitamins. The body must use water-soluble vitamins right away. Any leftover water-soluble vitamins leave the body through the urine. Vitamin B12 is the only water-soluble vitamin that can be stored in the liver for many years.

Calcium and Vitamin D Ineffective for Fractures, U.S. Preventive Services Task Force Says

Sunscreens and Vitamin D

Each of the vitamins listed below has an important job in the body. A vitamin deficiency occurs when you do not get enough of a certain vitamin. Vitamin deficiency can cause health problems.

Not eating enough fruits, vegetables, beans, lentils, whole grains and fortified dairy foods may increase your risk for health problems, including heart disease, cancer, and poor bone health (osteoporosis).

Vitamin A helps form and maintain healthy teeth, bones, soft tissue, mucus membranes, and skin.

Vitamin A is essential for reproduction and proper fetal development as well as strong vision and immune system function. Adult females need 700 micrograms of vitamin A daily, and adult males require 900 micrograms daily. Good food sources of vitamin A include organ meats, milk, cheese, eggs and fortified cereals.

Vitamin B6 is also called pyridoxine. Vitamin B6 helps form red blood cells and maintains brain function. This vitamin also plays an important role in the proteins that are part of many chemical reactions in the body. Eating larger amounts of protein may reduce vitamin B6 levels in the body.

Vitamin B12, like the other B vitamins, is important for metabolism. It also helps form red blood cells and maintains the central nervous system. There are a variety of vitamins that make up the category of B vitamins. Thiamin, riboflavin, niacin, B-6, pantothenic acid and biotin are co-enzymes, which mean they aid in a number of reactions that take place in the body. Folate and B-12 are required for the formation of red blood cells. Folate also contributes to neural development of a fetus.

Vitamin C, also called ascorbic acid, is an antioxidant that promotes healthy teeth and gums. It helps the body absorb iron and maintain healthy tissue. It also promotes wound healing. Vitamin C is necessary for bone, teeth, skin, blood vessel and immune system health. Although many people associate vitamin C with prevention of a cold, it does not actually prevent the cold but can reduce severity and length, according to "Nutrition & You." Men should consume 90 mg of vitamin C per day and women 75 mg. Most vitamin C is found in fruits and vegetables. Vitamin C, or ascorbic acid, is a water-soluble nutrient that can be found in citrus fruits, peppers, kiwi, broccoli, strawberries and cantaloupe. Vitamin C works as an antioxidant and prevents damage to the cells by free radicals. It is also essential for the body to make collagen, which can be found in your joints. The recommended daily allowance for vitamin C is 90 mg for adult men and 75 mg for adult women. A 2007 study published in the "The Journal of Bone and Joint Surgery" linked vitamin C to the reduction of complex regional pain syndrome in patients after wrist surgery. Researchers recommended a daily dose of at least 500 mg.

Vitamin D is also known as the "sunshine vitamin," since it is made by the body after being in the sun. Ten to 15 minutes of sunshine three times a week is enough to produce the body's requirement of vitamin D. People who do not live in sunny places may not make enough vitamin D. It is very difficult to get enough vitamin D from food sources alone. Vitamin D helps the body absorb calcium, which you need for the normal development and maintenance of healthy teeth and bones. It also helps maintain proper blood levels of calcium and phosphorus. Vitamin D is required for the proper absorption of phosphorous and calcium, which is needed for strong bones. Some research has shown vitamin D may also help prevent diabetes and some cancers, according to "Nutrition & You." Vitamin D can be synthesized from sunlight or consumed in fortified milk or cereals. Vitamin D is a fat-soluble nutrient that is essential to bone health as well as being connected to the prevention of autoimmune diseases like rheumatoid arthritis. It can be made naturally by exposing your skin to the ultraviolet B rays from the sun and is also found in fortified milk and salmon. The recommended daily allowance is 600 to 800 international units a day for adults.

Vitamin E is an antioxidant also known as tocopherol. It plays a role in the formation of red blood cells and helps the body use vitamin K. The most important function of vitamin E is as an antioxidant, which serves to protect the membranes of cells as well as prevent oxidation. Vitamin E also prevents the formation of blood clots. Adults should aim to consume 15 mg of vitamin E per day. Vitamin E is found in highest abundance in oils, nuts and seeds, but can also be found in leafy green vegetables and fortified cereals.

Vitamin K is not listed among the essential vitamins, but without it blood would not stick together (coagulate). Some studies suggest that it is important for promoting bone health. Vitamin K allows the blood to clot when necessary and plays a role in the synthesis of proteins that contribute to bone health. Adult women require 90 micrograms of vitamin K per day, and adult men require 120 micrograms per day. Green vegetables, such as broccoli, asparagus, spinach and brussels sprouts, are rich sources of vitamin K.

Biotin is essential for the metabolism of proteins and carbohydrates, and in the production of hormones and cholesterol.

Niacin is a B vitamin that helps maintain healthy skin and nerves. It is also has cholesterol-lowering effects.

Folate works with vitamin B12 to help form red blood cells. It is needed for the production of DNA, which controls tissue growth and cell function. Any woman who is pregnant should be sure to get enough folate. Low levels of folate are linked to birth defects such as spina bifida. Many foods are now fortified with folic acid.

Pantothenic acid is essential for the metabolism of food. It is also plays a role in the production of hormones and cholesterol.

Riboflavin (vitamin B2) works with the other B vitamins. It is important for body growth and the production of red blood cells.

Thiamine (vitamin B1) helps the body cells change carbohydrates into energy. Getting plenty of carbohydrates is very important during pregnancy and breast-feeding. It is also essential for heart function and healthy nerve cells.

.

FAT-SOLUBLE VITAMINS

Vitamin A:

Dark-colored fruit

Dark leafy vegetables

Egg yolk

Fortified milk and dairy products (cheese, yogurt, butter, and cream)

Liver, beef, and fish

Vitamin D:

Fish (fatty fish such as salmon, mackerel, herring, and orange roughy)

Fish liver oils (cod's liver oil)

Fortified cereals

Fortified milk and dairy products (cheese, yogurt, butter, and cream)

Vitamin E:

Avocado

Dark green vegetables (spinach, broccoli, asparagus, turnip greens)

Margarine (made from safflower, corn, and sunflower oil)

Oils (safflower, corn, and sunflower)

Papaya and mango

Seeds and nuts

Wheat germ and wheat germ oil

Vitamin K:

Cabbage

Cauliflower

Cereals

Dark green vegetables (broccoli, Brussels sprouts, asparagus)

Dark leafy vegetables (spinach, kale, collards, turnip greens)

Fish, liver, beef, eggs

WATER-SOLUBLE VITAMINS

Biotin:

Chocolate

Cereal

Egg yolk

Legumes

Milk

Nuts

Organ meats (liver, kidney)

Pork

Yeast

Folate:

Asparagus and broccoli

Beets

Brewer's yeast

Dried beans (cooked pinto, navy, kidney, and lima)

Fortified cereals

Green, leafy vegetables (spinach and romaine lettuce)

Lentils

Oranges and orange juice

Peanut butter

Wheat germ

Niacin (vitamin B3):

Avocado

Eggs

Enriched breads and fortified cereals

Fish (tuna and salt-water fish)

Lean meats

Legumes

Nuts

Potato

Poultry

Pantothenic acid:

Avocado

Broccoli, kale, and other vegetables in the cabbage family Eggs

Legumes and lentils

Milk

Mushroom

Organ meats

Poultry

White and sweet potatoes

Whole-grain cereals

Thiamine (vitamin B1):

Dried milk

Egg

Enriched bread and flour

Lean meats

Legumes (dried beans)

Nuts and seeds

Organ meats

Peas

Whole grains

Pyroxidine (vitamin B6):

Avocado

Banana

Legumes (dried beans)

Meat

Nuts

Poultry

Whole grains (milling and processing removes a lot of this vitamin)

Vitamin B12:

Meat

Eggs

Fortified foods such as soymilk

Milk and milk products

Organ meats (liver and kidney)

Poultry

Shellfish

NOTE: Animal sources of vitamin B13 are absorbed much better by the body than plant sources

Vitamin C (ascorbic acid):

Broccoli

Brussels sprouts

Cabbage

Cauliflower

Citrus fruits

Potatoes

Spinach

Strawberries

Tomato juice

Tomatoes

CALCIUM

What is calcium and what does it do?

Calcium is a mineral found in many foods. The body needs calcium to maintain strong bones and to carry out many important functions. Almost all calcium is stored in bones and teeth, where it supports their structure and hardness. Calcium also helps contract the muscles and dilate the blood vessels. Adults require 1,000 to 1,200 mg of calcium daily. Calcium is found in highest concentrations in milk, yogurt and cheese, but can also be found in broccoli, kale and salmon.

The body also needs calcium for muscles to move and for nerves to carry messages between the brain and everybody part. In addition, calcium is used to help blood vessels move blood throughout the body and to help release hormones and enzymes that affect almost every function in the human body.

How much calcium do I need?

The amount of calcium you need each day depends on your age. Average daily recommended amounts are listed below in milligrams (mg):

Birth to 6 months   200 mg

Infants 7–12 months 260 mg

Children 1–3 years 700 mg

Children 4–8 years 1,000 mg

Children 9–13 years 1,300 mg

Teens 14–18 years 1,300 mg

Adults 19–50 years 1,000 mg

Adult men 51–70 years 1,000 mg

Adult women 51–70 years 1,200 mg

Adults 71 years and older 1,200 mg

Pregnant and breastfeeding teens 1,300 mg

Pregnant and breastfeeding adults 1,000 mg

What foods provide calcium?

Calcium is found in many foods. You can get recommended amounts of calcium by eating a variety of foods, including the following:

•   Milk, yogurt, and cheese are the main food sources of calcium for the majority of people in the United States.

- Kale, broccoli, and Chinese cabbage are fine vegetable sources of calcium.

- Fish with soft bones that you eat, such as canned sardines and salmon, are fine animal sources of calcium.

- Most grains (such as breads, pastas, and unfortified cereals), while not rich in calcium, add significant amounts of calcium to the diet because people eat them often or in large amounts.

- Calcium is added to some breakfast cereals, fruit juices, soy and rice beverages, and tofu. To find out whether these foods have calcium, check the product labels.

What kinds of calcium dietary supplements are available?

Calcium is found in many multivitamin-mineral supplements, though the amount varies b by product. Dietary supplements that contain only calcium or calcium with other nutrients such as vitamin D are also available. Check the Supplement Facts label to determine the amount of calcium provided.

The two main forms of calcium dietary supplements are carbonate and citrate. Calcium carbonate is inexpensive, but is absorbed best when taken with food. Some over-the-counter antacid products, such as Tums® and Rolaids®, contain calcium carbonate. Each pill or chew provides 200–400 mg of calcium. Calcium citrate, a more expensive form of the supplement, is absorbed well on an empty or a full stomach. In addition, people with low levels of stomach acid (a condition more common in people older than 50) absorb calcium citrate more easily than calcium carbonate. Other forms of calcium in supplements and fortified foods include gluconate, lactate, and phosphate.

Calcium absorption is best when a person consumes no more than 500 mg at one time. So a person who takes 1,000 mg/day of calcium from supplements, for example, should split the dose rather than take it all at once.

Calcium supplements may cause gas, bloating, and constipation in some people. If any of these symptoms occur, try spreading out the calcium dose throughout the day, taking the supplement with meals, or changing the supplement brand or calcium form you take.

Am I getting enough calcium?

Many people don't get recommended amounts of calcium from the foods they eat, including:

- Girls aged 9 to 18 years,

- Women older than 50 years,

- Men older than 70 years.

However, when total calcium intakes from both food and supplements are considered, only adolescent girls still fall short of getting enough calcium, and some older women likely get more than the safe upper limit.

Certain groups of people are more likely than others to have trouble getting enough calcium:

- Postmenopausal women because they experience greater bone loss and do not absorb calcium as well. Sufficient calcium intake from food, and supplements if needed, can slow the rate of bone loss.

- Women of childbearing age whose menstrual periods stop (amenorrhea) because they exercise heavily, eat too little, or both. They need sufficient calcium to cope with the resulting decreased calcium absorption, increased calcium losses in the urine, and slowdown in the formation of new bone.

- People with lactose intolerance cannot digest this natural sugar found in milk and experience symptoms like bloating, gas, and diarrhea when they drink more than small amounts at a time. They usually can eat other calcium-rich dairy products that are low in lactose, such as yogurt and many cheeses, and drink lactose-reduced or lactose-free milk.

- Vegans (vegetarians who eat no animal products) and ovo-vegetarians (vegetarians who eat eggs but no dairy products), because they avoid the dairy products that are a major source of calcium in other people's diets.

Many factors can affect the amount of calcium absorbed from the digestive tract, including:

- Age. Efficiency of calcium absorption decreases as people age. Recommended calcium intakes are higher for people over age 70.

- Vitamin D intake. This vitamin, present in some foods and produced in the body when skin is exposed to sunlight, increases calcium absorption.

- Other components in food. Both oxalic acid (in some vegetables and beans) and phytic acid (in whole grains) can reduce calcium absorption. People who eat a variety of foods don't have to consider these factors. They are accounted for in the calcium recommended intakes, which take absorption into account.

Many factors can also affect how much calcium the body eliminates in urine, feces, and sweat. These include consumption of alcohol- and caffeine-containing beverages as well as intake of other nutrients (protein, sodium, potassium, and phosphorus). In most people, these factors have little effect on calcium status.

What happens if I don't get enough calcium?

Insufficient intakes of calcium do not produce obvious symptoms in the short term because the body maintains calcium levels in the blood by taking it from bone. Over the long term, intakes of calcium below recommended levels have health consequences, such as causing low bone mass (osteopenia) and increasing the risks of osteoporosis and bone fractures.

Symptoms of serious calcium deficiency include numbness and tingling in the fingers, convulsions, and abnormal heart rhythms that can lead to death if not corrected. These symptoms occur almost always in people with serious health problems or who are undergoing certain medical treatments.

What are some effects of calcium on health?

Bone health and osteoporosis

Bones need plenty of calcium and vitamin D throughout childhood and adolescence to reach their peak strength and calcium content by about age 30. After that, bones slowly lose calcium, but people can help reduce these losses by getting recommended amounts of calcium throughout adulthood and by having a healthy, active lifestyle that includes weight-bearing physical activity (such as walking and running).

Osteoporosis is a disease of the bones in older adults (especially women) in which the bones become porous, fragile, and more prone to fracture. Osteoporosis is a serious public health problem for more than 10 million adults in the United States. Adequate calcium and vitamin D intakes as well as regular exercise are essential to keep bones healthy throughout life.

High blood pressure

Some studies have found that getting recommended intakes of calcium can reduce the risk of developing high blood pressure (hypertension). One large study in particular found that eating a diet high in fat-free and low-fat dairy products, vegetables, and fruits lowered blood pressure.

Cancer

Studies have examined whether calcium supplements or diets high in calcium might lower the risks of developing cancer of the colon or rectum or increase the risk of prostate cancer. The research to date provides no clear answers. Given that cancer develops over many years, longer term studies are needed.

Kidney stones

Most kidney stones are rich in calcium oxalate. Some studies have found that higher intakes of calcium from dietary supplements are linked to a greater risk of kidney stones, especially among older adults. But calcium from foods does not appear to cause kidney stones. For most people, other factors (such as not drinking enough fluids) probably have a larger effect on the risk of kidney stones than calcium intake.

Weight loss

Although several studies have shown that getting more calcium helps lower body weight or reduce weight gain over time, most studies have found that calcium—from foods or dietary supplements—has little if any effect on body weight and amount of body fat.

Can calcium be harmful?

Getting too much calcium can cause constipation. It might also interfere with the body's ability to absorb iron and zinc, but this effect is not well established. In adults, too much calcium (from dietary supplements but not food) might increase the risk of kidney stones.

The safe upper limits for calcium are listed below. Most people do not get amounts above the upper limits from food alone; excess intakes usually come from the use of calcium supplements. Surveys show that some older women in the United States probably get amounts somewhat above the upper limit since the use of calcium supplements is common among these women.

Birth to 6 months   1,000 mg

Infants 7–12 months   1,500 mg

Children 1–8 years 2,500 mg

Children 9–18 years   3,000 mg

Adults 19–50 years   2,500 mg

Adults 51 years and older2,000 mg

Pregnant and breastfeeding teens   3,000 mg

Pregnant and breastfeeding adults   2,500 mg

Are there any interactions with calcium that I should know about?

Calcium dietary supplements can interact or interfere with certain medicines that you take, and some medicines can lower or raise calcium levels in the body. Here are some examples:

- Calcium can reduce the absorption of these drugs when taken together:

o   Bisphosphonates (to treat osteoporosis)

o   Antibiotics of the fluoroquinolone and tetracycline families

o   Levothyroxine (to treat low thyroid activity)

o   Phenytoin (an anticonvulsant)

o   Tiludronate disodium (to treat Paget's disease).

•   Diuretics differ in their effects. Thiazide-type diuretics (such as Diuril® and Lozol®) reduce calcium excretion by the kidneys which in turn can raise blood calcium levels too high. But loop diuretics (such as Lasix® and Bumex®) increase calcium excretion and thereby lower blood calcium levels.

•   Antacids containing aluminum or magnesium increase calcium loss in the urine.

•   Mineral oil and stimulant laxatives reduce calcium absorption.

•   Glucocorticoids (such as prednisone) can cause calcium depletion and eventually osteoporosis when people use them for months at a time.

Tell your doctor, pharmacist, and other health care providers about any dietary supplements and medicines you take. They can tell you if those dietary supplements might interact or interfere with your prescription or over-the-counter medicines or if the medicines might interfere with how your body absorbs, uses, or breaks down nutrients.

The body stores ninety percent of its calcium in the bones and teeth.

This huge percentage of calcium is not just stagnantly stored there and forgotten by the body. This storehouse of calcium is constantly used, replenished and washed through the system in a very minute molecular way. Some calcium molecules create a framework or nest for other calcium to come and go.

When you look at a bone that has osteoarthritis or osteoporosis, it looks porous, like a sponge. The center of the pore should be filled (and constantly replenished) with fine delicate calcium.

However, that skeletal calcium is the foundation of our house. How can you fix the foundation when there's a house on top of it? You have to repair the foundation and at the same time keep the house running.

Calcium is the third top biochemical foundation piece that makes up our body. The top four are: sodium, potassium, calcium, and magnesium. These four minerals act as the four corners of our foundation

Calcium is so important to keeping the body's biochemical balance that our body has very specific communication avenues just for calcium. These specific pathways run by osmosis, de-fusion, or active transport.

Bio-availability is Key to Calcium Metabolism

It is one thing to take calcium; it is another thing to take calcium in a form that is usable by the body. First it has to be absorbed within about the first twenty feet of the digestive tract, then absorbed into the blood stream and carried to the liver where is it reconstituted into a molecular form that is actually usable. The parathyroid takes it to the next step of usability.

Certain calcium molecules absorb slowly, some at a medium speed and some quickly. Each type has a different foundational function. The body requires many types of calcium to replenish the many different forms of calcium found in the body.

Every function, every organ and everything within the body relate to calcium in a specific way. Its primary function, from my point of view, is to alkalinize the body starting with the acid/alkaline balance of the digestive tract. All systems need a portion of the calcium to fully deal with aging, repairing and regenerating.

Solution To Calcium Replenishment

An ideal combination of different types of calcium would entirely replenish the empty or depleted stores that have been used by immune system to maintain balance as well as the long-term stores in the bones. Does such a product exist? Yes.

Of course, in order for the best metabolism of calcium, several other ingredients are needed, such as Vitamin D and magnesium. Vitamin D is needed, for the hormonal translation of calcium into calmodulin, calcitonin, calcitriol, calcidiol and cholcalciferol – all hormonal secondary molecules.

A natural source of magnesium is a rich chlorophyll product like alfalfa sprouts, liquid chlorophyll and Spirulina, or plants rich in magnesium, or water. Almonds are also a good source of both calcium and magnesium.

Different government studies over the years have shown that on average seventy-five percent of Americans are deficient in calcium. However digging a little deeper into that average, we find that women are more like 85% deficient and men are more like 65% deficient. So calcium deficiencies are an established fact, and more proof that our basic diet, with all the supposed "enriched with vitamins and minerals" isn't cutting it.

To paraphrase Einstein, if we keep eating and taking the same supplements the way we have been and yet expect different results, well, we are in for a surprise. Thus my focus on getting everyone to consciously take steps to get more, and a variety of, calcium into the diet.

The ideal Calcium supplement is food based and gives a number of different types of Calcium- gluconate, citrate and carbonate. These Herbal Calcium Tablets offer the necessary 1200 to 1400 mg's of calcium a day. Yes, the recommended daily requirement may not equal that amount, however from my studies of the effects of this formula, that is what I recommend. The benefits of using food-based Herbal Calcium Tablets is that the calcium absorption starts in the mouth's membranes (similar to a sub lingual), the calcium gets absorbed more readily and partly bypasses the losses that occur in the digestive tract to liver processing situation. The food-based source also helps correct the stomach acid/alkaline balance.

Expected Health Benefits of Herbal Calcium Tablets:

1. Clearer thinking: Calcium is used in our brain's biochemical action. Low calcium leads to memory loss as well as insomnia (can't stop thinking, restless brain symptoms).

2. Weight management and weight-loss: Yes weight management. Low calcium causes the body to go into an "I'm starving" mode that stimulates a hormone cascade that starts with the parathyroid releasing hormones, causing the bones to release calcium, causing the kidneys to release calcitriol to increase calcium absorption. This whole process also stimulates fat production and inhibits fat breakdown. High calcium intake stops the starvation cascade of hormones and its resultant fat production and preservation. (Ironically, with their high phosphoric acid content, diet sodas leach calcium from the body thus contributing to overweight conditions.)

3. Healthy teeth: Stands to reason, now that we know that our bones and teeth aren't set in stone but are in a constant state of coming and going.

4. Fewer PMS symptoms: Studies show improvement in both emotional and physical symptoms. (Maybe this should be reason #1).

5. Lowers risk of colon cancer: Scientists aren't sure of the exact mechanism, but studies find adequate to more than adequate intake of calcium has a protective effect.

6. Protection of your heart: That same starving hormone cascade that causes weight gain also affects your arteries. With an adequate supply of calcium your blood pressure gets reduced. Not the whole picture to heart health, but a simple and foundational step.

7. Natural relaxing mineral: Calcium relaxes muscles (no more Charlie horses) and aids in getting a better night's sleep. Just think how much better your days go when you get adequate sleep the night before and wake up all chipper!

8. Stronger immune system: Calcium is crucial to a healthy immune system.

Actions To Improve Calcium Uptake

Cut out drinks like sodas and coffee that, respectively, leach calcium or increase calcium excretion.

Eat more fruits and vegetables since the metabolizing of these foods shifts the acid/alkaline balance of the body towards an alkaline state by producing bicarbonate that reduces calcium loss. (Meat tends to cause the body to go acidic, thus causing the bones to release calcium and phosphorous).

Exercise improves calcium uptake. Maybe it is time to start dancing.

IRON

Iron is required for the proper formation of red blood cells as well as transport of oxygen to the tissues. Adult females require 18 mg of iron per day, adult males 8 mg. Iron is found in the greatest abundance in meat, poultry and fish. Grains and vegetables also provide small amounts of iron.

POTASSIUM

Potassium aids in many body functions including fluid balance, muscle contraction, nerve impulses, maintenance of blood pressure and bone health. Adults should aim to consume 4,700 mg of potassium per day. The U.S. Department of Agriculture notes that consuming an abundance of fruits and vegetables every day can help meet potassium needs easily.

Also listed are Herbs. For a long time I never really knew much about Herbs and what they could do for you. Since finding out about Herbs my life has changed a lot. Read on and see if you find out anything you never knew before.

HERBS for HEALING

Alfalfa

Family: Leguminosae Genus: Medicago Species: Sativa

Also Known As: Buffalo Grass, Chilean Clover

Alfalfa leaves have wonderful healing powers that can prevent heart disease, lower cholesterol and help prevent strokes.

Warnings: Alfalfa seeds should never be ingested as they contain high levels of amino acid canavanine. Some chemicals in alfalfa can also destroy red blood cells and people with anemia should use caution when ingesting it.

Allspice

Family: Myrtaceae Genus: Pimenta Species: Officinalis, Dioca

Also Known As: Clove Pepper, Pimento, Pimenta, Jamaican Pepper

Rx: cooking, oil for toothache, infusion for digestive aid

Allspice is used as a digestive aid, anesthetic, and pain reliever and has been used to treat flatulence and diabetes.

Warnings:Allspice oil should never be swallowed as it can cause nausea, vomiting, and even convulsions. The oil can also be irritating when applied externally to people with sensitive skin or those with eczema.

Aloe

Family: Liliaceae Genus: Aloe Species: Vera (and over 500 others)

Also Known As: Socotrine, Cape, Curaiao, Barbados, Zanzibar Aloe

Rx: cut mature (lower) leaves for burns, scalds, sunburns, or cosmetic benefits

Aloe is one of the most widely used herbs for burns, scalds, scrapes, sunburn, and an incredible infection fighter. It can also be used to smooth and beautify skin.

Warnings:Aloe latex is a very powerful laxative and may cause severe cramps and diarrhea. It should never be ingested by pregnant women as it may cause miscarriage.

Anise

Family: Umbelliferae Genus: Pimpinella Species: Anisum

Also Known As: Aniseed, Sweet Cumin

Rx: infusion of seeds, tinctures

It has been used as a cough remedy, digestive aid, and contains chemicals similar to estrogen, which may help with menopausal discomforts, and has been known to treat some cases of prostate cancer.

Warnings:If your doctor has advised you not to use birth control pills then you should seek the advise of a physician before using this herb because it contains estrogen.

Balm, Lemon

Family: Labiatae Genus: Melissa Species: Officinalis

Also Known As: Bee Balm, Balm, Sweet Balm, Melissa, Cure-all

Rx: leaves in bath, compress for wounds, infusion, tincture

You can use it to treat wounds, herpes, viral infections, and has been used as a digestive aid, and a tranquilizer. It can also be used to treat menstrual cramps or to promote menstruation.

Warnings:Anyone with a thyroid condition should avoid using this herb because it contains a thyroid-stimulating hormone, thyrotropin.

Basil

Family: Labiatae Genus: Ocimum Species: Basilicum, Sanctum

Also Known As: Sweet Basil, St. Josephwort

Rx: tincture or infusion for acne and general infection fighting

It has been used to treat intestinal parasites, acne, and stimulates the immune system.

Warnings: Tests have shown that basil may contain a chemical that has caused liver tumors in mice, although the cancer risks remain unclear and not even the most conservative herb critics advise caution when using it.

Bay

Family: Lauraceae Genus: Laurus Species: Nobilis

Also Known As: Sweet Bay, Green Bay, Laurel, Grecian or Roman Laurel

Rx: fresh leaves for wounds, infusion, tincture

Bay is not only used as a bug repellent, but has been known to soothe sore joints, treat infections, and when added to a bath may help with relaxation.

Warnings:External uses of bay should be avoided if you have sensitive skin as it may cause a rash.

Caraway

Family: Umbelliferae Genus: Caurm Species: Carvi

Also Known As: Carum

Rx: seeds in food, oil, infusion of seeds, tincture

Two chemicals in caraway seeds have been known to soothe the digestive tract and to help expel gas. It may also be used for relief of menstrual cramps due to the fact that caraway might relax the uterus.

Catnip

Family: Labiatae Genus: Nepeta Species: Cataria

Also Known As: Catnep, Catswort, Catmint, Field Balm

Rx: infusion of flowers and leaves (for you not your cat!)

When used in teas, it is considered a cold and cough remedy because it relieves chest congestion and loosens phlegm. Catnip has long been used as a sedative, tranquilizer, digestive aid, menstruation promoter, and treatment for menstrual cramps, flatulence, and infant colic.

Warnings: Some people may experience upset stomach but Catnip is considered nontoxic.

Chamomile

Family: Compositae Genus: Matricaria, Anthemis Species: Chamomilla, Nobilis respectively

Also Known As: Camomile, Anthemis, Matricaria, Ground Apple

Rx: infusion or tincture of flowers, herbal bath

This herb is a highly used cure-all, and every household should seriously consider having it around. It has been used externally to treat wounds and inflammations, and internally for indigestion and ulcers. Chamomile is also used to relieve menstrual cramps, arthritis, and is an effective sedative.

Warnings: People who have previously suffered anaphylactic reactions from ragweed should think twice about using this herb as well as its close relative yarrow. Large amounts have caused some nausea and vomiting.

Chicory

Family: Compositae Genus: Cicorium Species: Intybus

Also Known As: Endive, Chickory

Rx: excellent salad addition, infusion, tincture

It is also known as endive, or chickory. Chicory is most commonly used to reduce the bitter taste of caffeine in coffee. It aids in cleansing the urinary tract, digestion, a mild laxative and is also taken for rheumatic conditions and gout. Many times I have added this to my ground coffee and it sure does work. Much more mellow coffee.

Cinnamon

Family: Lauraceae Genus: Cinnamomum Species: Zeylanicum, Cassia, Saigonicum

Also Known As: Ceylon Cinnamon, Saigon Cinnamon, Cassia

Rx: infusion of powdered herb, sprinkle cuts or scrapes for treatment

Cinnamon

About 5 years ago, we heard from a reader that cinnamon might help lower blood sugar in someone with type 2 diabetes. That was news to us, but a little sleuthing did turn up some interesting animal cell research. Studies showed that cinnamon made cells more responsive to insulin, which theoretically would lead to better glucose control. Since then we have heard from many readers that a little cinnamon does indeed help them keep their blood sugar in check.

Cinnamon lowers blood sugar and cholesterol. People usually enjoy the taste of cinnamon when it's added to apple cider or baked goods. Putting a small amount of cinnamon in foods or taking cinnamon in capsules can significantly improve blood-sugar levels. Be warned, though: eating a Cinnabon, which has 144 grams of sugars and carbs and 730 calories, won't do anything good for you. Researchers at the U.S. Department of Agriculture and their counterparts from Pakistan tested the effects of cinnamon-containing capsules on 60 people with diabetes.

Cinnamon has been shown to reduce lipids and have anti-inflammatory and platelet-adhesion properties. The results of a study demonstrated that intake of small amounts of cinnamon per day (no more than six grams or one-fifth of an ounce) reduced serum glucose, triglyceride, LDL cholesterol, and total cholesterol in people with type 2 diabetes. In an animal study, male rats who were given an extract of cinnamon had lower blood glucose levels. A human study found that giving cinnamon extract to type 2 diabetics significantly reduced their blood sugar levels.

Cinnamon is an insulin substitute in Type II diabetes. Cinnamon itself has insulin-like activity, increasing the effectiveness of insulin. Cinnamon also has a bio-active component that has the potential to prevent or overcome diabetes. It also increases vitality, balances energy, improves the digestion of fruits, milk, and other dairy products and helps reduce bloating and gas. Where to buy it: At the grocery store. If you have access to purchasing on line, you can purchase cinnamon in bulk very inexpensively.

You can get a pound of cinnamon for less than $5, and save yourself dreadful side effects. Cinnamon helps to control blood sugar levels in type 2 diabetics. Ground cinnamon helps stimulate the production of glucose-burning enzymes and boosts insulin's effectiveness. In one study, cinnamon made insulin 20 times more capable of breaking down blood sugars.

For hundreds of years, the ancient Greeks and Romans used cinnamon for better digestion. Although scientists can't tell you how it works, it might have to do with the way cinnamon heats up your stomach. Whatever the reason, adding some cinnamon to your meal could help relieve your discomfort if you have trouble with frequent indigestion. If you have adult-onset diabetes, talk with your doctor about using cinnamon in your diet. Test tube studies showed that a pinch of cinnamon can make insulin work better.

Cinnamon is used for infection prevention, pain relief, a digestive aid, and may help calm the uterus.

Warnings: Do not ingest cinnamon oil. It can cause nausea, vomiting, and possible kidney damage. When put on the skin, the oil may cause redness and burning.

How does cinnamon and weight loss work?

How is cinnamon and weight loss related? Well, it has to do with how the body uses insulin, which is a substance (hormone) produced by the body that's needed for the metabolism/use of carbohydrate for energy production.

Insulin is the hormone that tells the cells in your body to accept glucose (broken down carbohydrate) so that it can be used for energy. It also signals the body to store any fat for later use since there is carbohydrate to hand that is being used for energy.

However, the body can develop a resistance to insulin from poor nutrition, lack of physical activity, toxic build-up and other causes. Cells then resist the insulin, basically becoming jammed or clogged, and can't use the glucose in the blood stream. The level of glucose thus increases in the blood stream and we get the condition of type 2 diabetes.

What does the body do then? Well, it starts pumping even more insulin into the body in an attempt to lower the glucose that's now piling up in the blood because it's not getting into the cells.

The person starts craving and eating more carbohydrate to try and handle his lack of energy - but because of the insulin resistance, the fuel (glucose) from the carbohydrate hardly gets into his cells. So the vicious cycle continues with more and more insulin being pumped into the body but not being well used.

Remember that insulin also tells the body to store fat instead of use it since there is already fuel from the carbohydrate.

So we get a situation where the body actually can't burn fat for fuel.

Here's the great news about cinnamon and weight loss! Cinnamon helps the body to utilize insulin properly, reducing insulin resistance.

One half teaspoon before each of 3 meals plus one half teaspoon before bedtime is recommended. You can sprinkle it on foods, add it to tea, whatever you like to use it with.

Maybe you've realized while reading this that if you're consuming a lot of carbohydrate (not difficult if you're eating packaged and processed food, fast food and other "junk food") that the more carbohydrate you give your body, the less fat it will use for energy.

So if you're considering using cinnamon and weight loss is the reason, it's vital to understand that cinnamon alone isn't a "magic pill" that will help you lose weight. It may very well help your body to lose weight when you combine it with healthy eating, drinking enough water, a bit of physical activity and enough sleep!

Clove

Family: Myrtaceae Genus: Eugenia, Syzygium Species: Caryophyllata, Aromaticum respectively

Also Known As: Caryophyllus, Clavos

Rx: oil for toothache, infusion

It has been used for toothaches, oral hygiene, a digestive aid, and an infection fighter. It is also used to treat hernia, ringworm, and athlete's foot.

Warnings: Children under the age of 2 should never be given clove for medicinal purposes. The oil may cause stomach upset when swallowed, and used externally may cause rash.

Coriander

Family: Umbelliferae Genus: Corinadrum Species: Sativum

Also Known As: Cilantro, Chinese Parsley

Rx: infusion of seeds, sprinkle on cuts and scrapes

Used for indigestion, flatulence, and diarrhea, and externally for muscles and joint pains.

Warnings: If Coriander causes minor discomforts, such as stomach upsets or diarrhea, use less or stop using it.

Cranberry

Family: Ericaceae Genus: Vaccinium, Oxycoccus Species: Macerocarpon, Quadripetalus respectively

Also Known As: N/A

Rx: Juice, juice, juice!

Used for urinary tract infections (UTI), incontinence, high Vitamin C content

Dandelion

Family: Compositae Genus: Taraxacum Species: Officinale

Also Known As: Wild Endive, Lion's Tooth, Piss-in-bed

Rx: #1 recommended salad addition, leaf infusion, root decoction, tincture, add to bath for prevention of yeast infection

Used for Premenstrual Syndrome (PMS), Weight Loss, High Blood Pressure, Congestive Heart Failure, Cancer Prevention, Yeast Infection, Digestive Aid

Eat fresh leaves in a salad (they are quite tasty). Chinese doctors have prescribed Dandelion for thousands of years to treat colds, bronchitis, pneumonia, ulcers, hepatitis, obesity, dental problems, itching and internal injuries. Quite simply a 'super' herb.

As one of the most used herbs in herbal medicine traditions all over the world, dandelion is especially known for the health benefits it provides for the liver. Along
with milk thistle and burdock root, dandelion is one of the most recommended herbs
for liver detoxification. Since the liver's primary function is to detoxify every chemical, pollutant and medicine that the body is exposed to, it is essential that it stays healthy so it can function efficiently. Dandelion is often used as a remedy for hepatitis C. Both dandelion root and dandelion leaves can be used to detoxify the liver and keep it in good health.

Dandelion is a mild choleretic, which means that it stimulates the release of bile from
the liver into the gallbladder. Dandelion is used to support treatment of a variety of liver and gallbladder disorders, especially the incomplete digestion of fats. One of the
active compounds in dandelion is called taraxacin, which stimulates the liver and gallbladder to release bile. The release of bile is useful in constipation and indigestion
since bowels move more easily with increased bile flow. Bile also helps with the absorption and digestion of fats. Another health benefit of dandelion is that it's a natural diuretic. Dandelion stimulates urination but also replaces the potassium lost due to the increased volume of urine. Due to its diuretic properties, dandelion is one
of the best remedies for reducing high blood pressure. (Consult with your physician
before discontinuing use of blood pressure medications.) Dandelion leaves are an excellent addition to salad greens or they can be eaten alone. Dandelion roots can be prepared like carrots and added to stir-fries, soups, or sautéed with onions and garlic. The root is often used to make a liver detoxifying tea with either just dandelion root or a blend of dandelion root and other herbs.
Warnings: May cause skin rash in sensitive cases. If Dandelion causes stomach upset or diarrhea, use less or stop using it.

Dandelion is one of the best herbs for cleansing and detoxification with laxative and diuretic properties. Europeans have used dandelion for anemia, diabetes and liver disease.

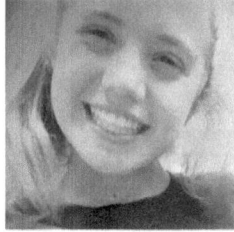

Just think of all the Dandelions you have in your yard. We pick them each year and throw them away and yet they are so valuable for our health. Next time you see a dandelion, don't look at it as a week that ruins your lawn .. look at it as a herb that will benefit your body in so many ways. I have drank Dandelion Tea now for about two years and actually feel the benefit of it. Having rheumatoid Arthritis has been a real draw back for me, but since drinking the tea the pain and movement in my joints have subsided considerably.

The directions here are for the do-it-yourselfer, but you can also purchase bags of chopped dandelion roots in your local Health Food Store.

How to dry your own dandelion roots

1.   Harvest Dandelion Roots in the fall after flowering, although any time is fine.

2.   Wash the roots well and dry.

3.   Crush them into pieces the best you can or slice thinly.

4.   Spread the dandelion roots on a baking pan or dehydrator rack

5.   Bake at a very low temperature (200 – 250 degrees) and bake until they are dry, or dehydrate until dry – it may take a long time. If baking in the oven, leave the oven door open slightly so the moisture can escape. Stir occasionally to make sure the roots are drying evenly. Cool.

6.   Store dried dandelion roots in an airtight container/package.

Directions for dandelion tea

Ingredients:

•   1 tablespoon of dried roots

•   1 cup of hot water

Let steep for 5 minutes.

Drink dandelion tea hot or cold.

Dill

Family: Umbelliferae Genus: Anethum Species: Graveolens

Also Known As: N/A

Rx: chew seed for fresh breath, infusion or tincture, add to bath to for prevention of urinary tract infections

In addition to its preservative action, Dill is an infection fighter and soothing digestive aid. Used for stomach problems, flatulence, urinary tract infection (UTI)

Warnings: May cause skin rash in sensitive individuals.

Echinacea

Family: Compositae Genus: Echinacea Species: Angustifolia, Purpurea

Also Known As: Coneflower, Purple Coneflower

Rx: tincture or decoction of the ROOTS

The best kept secret of the west. This is our A#1 recommended herb due to its high immune system boost. Echinacea kills a wide variety of disease causing viruses and bacteria, it fights infection and strengthens tissues. It may prevent infection by seriously boosting ones immune system. It is known to help the body in fighting off colds and flu. It is a treatment for yeast infections and actually can reduce the future onset of. It helps preserve white blood cells, is a confirmed wound healer as it prevents germs from penetrating tissues, and may have anti-arthritic properties. It is simply the most productive herb off all time.

Warnings:often causes one's tongue to tingle, this is not harmful.

Eucalyptus

Family: Myrtaceae Genus: Eucalyptus Species: Globulus

Also Known As: Gum Tree, Blue Gum, Australian Fever Tree

Rx: boil leaves as an inhalant, oil on cuts and scrapes, infusion from leaves NOT OIL, add leaves to bath

Eucalyptol is the chemical that gives Eucalyptus its healing properties. It loosens phlegm, kills influenza, and may help bacterial bronchitis. An effective treatment for minor cuts and scrapes and it even repels cockroaches!

Warnings:Do NOT ingest Eucalyptus oil, it is highly poisonous. Fatalities have been reported from ingestion of as little as a teaspoon. KEEP AWAY FROM CHILDREN!

Fennel

Family: Umbelliferae Genus: Foeniculum Species: Vulgare, Vulgare Dulce

Also Known As: Finocchio, Carosella, Florence Fennel

Rx: chew seeds for a digestive aid, infusion, tincture

Fennel relaxes the smooth muscle lining of the digestive tract and also helps expel gas. Used in Germany for infant colic. Traditionally used to stimulate the uterus into menstruation. This herb may also help fight prostate cancer.

Warnings:Since Fennel has a mild estrogenic effect, do not use if you are currently taking birth control pills, have a history of abnormal blood clotting, or estrogen dependent breast tumors. Do NOT ingest Fennel Oil, seeds are fine but the oil may cause nausea, vomiting, and possibly seizures.

Feverfew

Family: Compositae Genus: Chrysanthemum, Matricaria, Tanacetum Species: Parthenium

Also Known As: Ferbrifuge Plant, Wild Quinine, Bachelor's Button

Rx: chew leaves for migraine control, premade pills and tablets also work well for headaches, infusion, tincture

Got a headache, maybe a chronic migraine? Feverfew may well be your answer. Seventy percent of patients in scientific studies show a significant improvement in their migraine headaches even when standard medical treatment showed no results. Also traditionally used for gynecological purposes. This herb may reduce high blood pressure, and is a great digestive aid after meals.

Warnings:may cause sores inside the mouth, do not take if you have a clotting disorder. Remember that Feverfew does not CURE migraines, it suppresses them.

Ginger

Family: Zingiberaceae Genus: Zingiber Species: Officinale

Also Known As: Asian, African, American Ginger

Rx: cooking, capsules for motion sickness; tea, infusion, or ginger-ale for digestive aid.

This herb helps with motion and morning sickness. It is a very good digestive aid, may ease menstrual cramps, helps arthritis, is traditionally used in the orient for colds and flu, and is excellent for reducing cholesterol, lowering blood pressure, and preventing internal blood clots (heart attacks)

Ginger Detox Bath

Another alternative to a detox bath is to add 1/8 cup of freshly grated ginger to your bath. Ginger is wonderful for detoxing the body, opening the pores of your skin and eliminating toxins.

To enhance the effectiveness of an Epsom salts or ginger detox, make sure you drink 2 glasses of water before and after the bath. You can also gain added benefit by wrapping yourself in a towel after rubbing yourself vigorously and while you are still warm put yourself under the bed covers and try to fall asleep. You will continue to sweat for a good hour or so afterwards which will further release toxins.

Warnings:large doses MIGHT cause a miscarriage although there are no scientific reports backing this up.

Ginkgo

Family: Ginkgoaceae Genus: Ginkgo Species: Biloba

Also Known As: Maidenhair Tree

Rx: leaves brewed as tea, infusion

The Earth's oldest tree, it's a given that this herb helps the elderly the most. Ginkgo increases blood flow to the brain which can prevent strokes and heart attacks, improve memory, help impotence and chronic dizziness. It is also known to help with macular degeneration (blindness), circulation, asthma, tinnitus, and deafness. A fine example of the need to preserve the Earth's natural resources.

Warnings:Do not use if you have a clotting disorder, do not take in very large amounts as diarrhea, vomiting, and irritability can occur.

Ginseng

Family: Araliaceae Genus: Panax, Eleutherococcus Species: Ginseng and Quinquefolius, Senticosus

Also Known As: Root of Immortality, Man Root, Life Root, Seng Seng

Rx: It is very important to use mature roots (over 6 years old). Use root powder teas, capsules or tablets. You can also make a decoction from dried pulverized root.

This herb helps the bodies resistance, boosts the immune system, lowers cholesterol, lowers blood sugars, reduces heart attacks, protects the liver, helps the appetite, and helps cancer patients with radiation therapy.

Warnings:Rare cases of insomnia, allergy symptoms, breast soreness. Do not use if you have high blood pressure, fever, asthma, emphysema, or cardiac arrhythmia.

Horehound

Family: Labiatae Genus: Marrubium Species: Vulgare

Also Known As: Marrubium, Hoarhound, White Horehound

Rx: flowers and leaves in infusion or tincture for cough remedy

A popular herbal cough remedy and expectorant for almost 2,000 years, Horehound is good for minor respiratory problems, coughs, colds, and bronchitis

Warnings:those with heart disease should not use this herb

Hyssop

Family: Labiatae Genus: Hyssopus Species: Officinalis

Also Known As: N/A

Rx: flowers and leaves as a compress for cold sores and genital herpes, infusion, tincture

Hyssop inhibits the growth of herpes simplex virus. Scientists agree it is a 'reasonably effective' treatment for cough and irritation of colds and flu.

Warnings:DO NOT USE IF PREGNANT..... PERIOD! Again always positively identify the herbs you use. H. Officinalis is the correct herb, it's name sharing cousins (G. Officinalis, genus' Agastache and Bacopa) should not be ingested.

Juniper

Family: Cupressaceae Genus: Juniperus Species: Communis

Also Known As: Geneva, Genvrier

Rx: infusion of berries for arthritis or female regularity

The source of gin, this herb also increases urine production (a diuretic) - making it a treatment for PMS, high blood pressure and congestive heart failure. Recommended for arthritis.

Warnings:Long term use can cause kidney damage. If you have a kidney infection or kidney problems you should not use this herb. One-third of hay fever sufferers develop allergy symptoms from exposure to Juniper.

Kelp

Family: Fucaceae Genus: Fucus, Laminaria, Macrocystis, Nereocystis Species: Versiculosus (Fucus), various (Others)

Also Known As: Fucus, Seawrack, Cutweed, Bladderwrack, Wakame, Hijiki, Kombu, Arame

A natural source of iodine, now known as a radiation protector, protection from heavy metals, reducer of heart disease, and an infection fighter.

Rx: take tablets (herb is unpleasant), infusion

Warnings: None

Lavender

Genus: Lavendula Species: Angustifolia

Also Known As: English Lavender

Rx: flowers in bath, general aromatherapy

The all time fragrant herb, Lavender makes a great bath addition. The Greeks and Romans bathed in lavender scented water and it was from the Latin word, lavo (to wash) that the herb took its name. While not technically a medicinal herb, the calming properties of its aroma are well founded.

Warnings: None

Marijuana

Genus: Cannabis Species: Sativa, Indica, others

Also Known As: Weed, Cannabis, Pot, Dope

The much debated and scolded Cannabis, Marijuana has shown positive effects on cancer, AIDS, and glaucoma. So effective on AIDS patients from its ability to increase a person's appetite as well as releiving nausea allowing a patient to regain weight. Marijuana reportedly helps glaucoma patients by reducing occular pressure which can cause damage to the eye. It is the most effective treatment for chronic nausea. It is not physically addictive.

Rx: smoked (dried), added to salads(fresh)

Warnings: coughing, asthma, upper respiratory problems, difficulty with short term memory loss, racing heart, agitation, confusion, paranoia, possible psychological dependence

Marjoram

Family: Labiatae Genus: Origanum Species: Majorana, others

Also Known As: Oregano(many palates cannot tell the difference!), Knotted Marjoram

Rx: sprinkle dried powdered herb on cold sores or genital herpes, infusion or tincture for its stomach soothing potential

An excellent digestive aid and herpes fighter, this one of the most confused herbs on the planet. The Oregano on your spice rack might be Marjoram! All Marjoram species are called Oregano but only a few of the fifty are ever called Marjoram.

Warnings:None

Mint

Family: Labiatae Genus: Mentha Species: Piperita (Peppermint), Cardiaca (Spearmint), Spicata, Viridis, Aquatica

Also Known As: Numerous kinds of mint

Rx: Peppermint oil for wounds, burns etc., infusion of any dried mint for decongestant, tincture

The after dinner mint soothes the stomach. Peppermint produces Menthol. Menthol is a key anesthetic (e.g. Ben-Gay), the vapors are an incredible decongestant (e.g. Vick's VapoRub), is germicidal, and helps morning sickness a great deal. Those wishing to alleviate morning sickness should use only dilute tea concentrations for reasons shown below. Peppermint is a hybrid of Spearmint and is the more potent due to the high menthol factor. Spearmint contains Carvone in comparison to Menthol. While not nearly as effective, Spearmint is much safer.

Warnings:on rare occasions the fragrance of mint oil has caused gagging in children. Pure Menthol, ingested, is POISONOUS. A teaspoon can be FATAL. DO NOT ingest Peppermint oil or Menthol.

Mistletoe

Family: Loranthaceae Genus: Viscum, Phoradendron Species: Album, Serotinum

Also Known As: Lignum Crucis, Herbe de la Croix, Viscum

Rx: leaves in DILUTED infusion, tincture for high blood pressure

Mistletoe, the kissing plant, has the ability to slow the pulse, lower blood pressure and stimulate gastrointestinal and uterine contractions.

Warnings:should be administered only by a qualified herbal/medicinal doctor. TWO BERRIES CAN KILL A CHILD. Keep away from children. This herb is highly toxic. Pregnant women should not use it. This herb is known (unfortunately) for its abortion inducing properties.

The dose needed to induce abortion is enough to kill you.

Myrrh

Family: Burseraceae Genus: Commiphora Species: Abyssinica, Myrrha

Also Known As: Balsamodendron

Rx: steep powdered herb for mouthwash, infusion, tincture

Myrrh makes an excellent mouthwash, toothpaste, and fights bacteria

Warnings:large amounts may have violent laxative action

Nettle

Family: Urticaceae Genus: Urtica Species: Dioica

Also Known As: Stinging Nettle, Common Nettle, Greater Nettle

Rx: process plant matter in juicer, infusion, tincture

An effective cure for gout, Nettle is also good for the symptoms of hay fever, scurvy, PMS, and helps heart patients.

Warnings:When I was a child, I must have fallen into Nettle a hundred times. USE THICK GLOVES. If you doubt the cruelty of natures own protections just touch one of these plants. Large doses of Nettle tea may cause stomach irritation.

Oregano (see Marjoram)

Parsley

Family: Umbelliferae Genus: Petroselinum Species: Crispum, Hortense, Sativum

Also Known As: Rock Selinon

Rx: a few sprigs for fresh breath, infusion of leaves and seeds, tincture

The seeds and the leaves of this plant contain the oil that is known to curb high blood pressure, help with fever, freshen breath, help with allergies and help heart patients.

Warnings: do not use to promote weight loss

Pepper, Red

Family: Solanaceae Genus: Capsicum Species: Annuum, Frutescens

Also Known As: Hot pepper, most of the pepper family including bell pepper

Rx: cooking, infusion

It is a good digestive aid, can relieve infectious diarrhea (and can bring on noninfectious diarrhea if too many hot peppers are ingested), helps chronic pain when used externally, is the best shingles reliever, helps headaches, and tastes great!

Warnings: can burn the eyes, mouth and skin

Rosemary

Family: Labiatae Genus: Rosmarinus Species: Officinalis

Also Known As: Rosemarine, Incensier

Rx: cooking, excellent tea, infusion, tincture

In ancient times people wrapped their meat with Rosemary to prevent spoilage. Rosemary is a natural preservative. Rosemary can prevent food poisoning, is a digestive aid, is a good decongestant and can kill bacteria. If you enjoy using Rosemary in your cooking, use more.

Warnings: do not ingest Rosemary oil, in large amounts, poisoning can occur

Saffron

Family: Iridaceae Genus: Crocus Species: Sativus

Also Known As: Spanish Saffron

Rx: 12 to 15 stigmas per cup of boiling water

Since it takes 75,000 flowers to make one pound of Saffron, this herb is very expensive. Heart attack patients may actually save money using this as it is much cheaper than some clot dissolving drugs injected to treat heart attack. It can help to control some risk factors for heart disease. It also reduces cholesterol, de-clogs the arteries, and lowers blood pressure.

Warnings: unless you are pregnant, just the high cost

Sage

Family: Labiatae Genus: Salvia Species:Officinalis

Also Known As: All types of Sage

Rx: crushed fresh leaves for cuts and wounds, infusion of dried leaves, tincture

Sage is the premiere anti-perspirant, cutting perspiration by up to 50 percent. It is a great fighter against infection, a good preservative, a digestive aid, can reduce blood sugar and helps a sore throat! And its flavor in meats and sausage is unrivaled.

Warnings: rare cases of inflammation of the lips and lining of the mouth. Sage oil should not be ingested.

Savory

Family: Labiatae Genus: Satureja Species: Hortensis, Montana

Also Known As: White Thyme, Bean Herb

A great culinary herb, Savory has great soothing properties for children, it is a great expectorant and digestive aid and is subtle enough for use with children.

Rx: infusion of leaves for childhood colds

Warnings: None

Skullcap

Family: Labiatae Genus: Scutellaria Species: Lateriflora

Also Known As: Quaker Bonnet, Mad Dog Weed, Hoodwort, Helmet Flower

Rx: use leaf infusion for tranquilizing effects

European medical experts now accept skullcap's potential usefulness as a tranquilizer and sedative, and it is used in many commercial sleep preparations that are widely available in Europe.

Warnings: large doses may result in confusion, giddiness, twitching, and possible convulsions

Tarragon

Family: Compositae Genus: Artemisia Species: Dracunculus

Also Known As: Dragon Herb, Estragon, French or Russian Tarragon

Rx: chew fresh leaves for toothache, apply fresh leaves to cuts and wounds, infusion of leaves, tincture

A wonderful treatment for toothache, Tarragon is a great anesthetic and prevents infections.

Warnings: those with history of Cancer should not use this herb

Tea

Family: Theaceae Genus: Camellia Species: Sinensis

Also Known As: Green Tea, Black Tea

Rx: typical leaf infusion

From the Orient, to the United Kingdom, Tea is widely used for its calming effects. Tea includes stimulants that help colds, congestion, asthma, diarrhea, tooth decay and helps prevent tissue damage from radiation therapy. Tea only grows in India, Sri Lanka, and Indonesia and is imported around the world. Green Tea is simply the dried leaf, Black Tea is dried and then fermented.

Warnings: Caffeine addiction, problems associated with Caffeine

Thyme

Family: Labiatae Genus: Thymus Species: Vulgaris, Serpyllum

Also Known As: Mother of Thyme, Common or Garden Thyme, Wild, Creeping or Mother Thyme

As well as a culinary delight, Thyme fights several disease causing bacteria and viruses. It is a good digestive aid, helps menstrual cramps and is a great cough remedy. Germany uses it today to treat whoop, whooping cough and emphysema.

Rx: fresh leaves for cuts and wounds, tincture for antiseptic, infusion of leaves for the stomach, cough or menstrual symptoms.

Warnings: Do not ingest Thyme oil, it can lead to headache, nausea, vomiting, weakness, thyroid impairment, and heart and respiratory depression.

Valerian

Family: Valerianaceae Genus: Valeriana Species: Officinalis

Also Known As: Phu, Heal-all, Garden Valerian

Rx: infusion of root for sedative properties, tincture

The quite smelly and pungent Valerian is a powerful sedative that was even listed as a tranquilizer in the National Formulary until 1950. A great replacement for users of valium, Valerian can also reduce high blood pressure.

Warnings: large doses may cause headache, giddiness, blurred vision, restlessness, nausea, and morning grogginess.

Vervain

Family: Verbenaceae Genus: Verbena Species: Officinalis, Hastata

Also Known As: Indian Hyssop, Blue Vervain, Verbena, Enchanter's Herb

Rx: infusion of leaves for headache and arthritis, tincture

'Take two Vervain and call me in the morning' is how it should be said. Vervain is a great substitute for aspirin as it has similar effects. Vervain outside of being a very mild laxative is mainly used for mild pain relief.

Warnings: anyone with a history of heart problems should not use this herb

Witch Hazel

Family: Hamamelidaceae Genus: Hamamelis Species: Virginiana

Also Known As: Hamamelis, Snapping Hazelnut, Winterbloom

Rx: astringent decoction of leaves and twigs, astringent gargle

A primary astringent in the herbal world, Witch Hazel has antiseptic, anesthetic, astringent, and anti-inflammatory properties. The clear, pungent extract is a standard for cuts, bruises, hemorrhoids, and sore muscles. It is one of this nation's most widely used healing herbs. It is much better to find fresh Witch Hazel than rely on commercial products containing it.

Warnings: may be used externally on anyone but dilute for children.

GARLIC

Garlic

Family: Amaryllidacae Genus: Allium Species: Sativum

Also Known As: Stinking Rose, Heal-all, Poor Man's Treacle

Rx: use cloves in cooking, crush and encapsulate or use premade tablets, infusion.

Garlic is the world's second oldest medicine, and is the traditional 'WONDER DRUG'. Many people don't realize that onion has almost as much medicinal value as garlic does. Battle wounds in WWI were treated with garlic juice. Recommended for colds, coughs, flu, fever, bronchitis, ringworm, intestinal worms, elevated cholesterol, and general internal organ problems. No standard medication can match Garlic on the cardiovascular scale. Garlic DEFINITELY reduces blood pressure, cholesterol, and reduces internal clots which can lead to heart attacks and stroke. Garlic reduces blood sugar and therefore helps diabetes sufferers. It may help eliminate lead and heavy metals in the bloodstream, has helped leprosy patients, fights cancer, helps AIDS patients.

Warnings: Allergy sufferers may develop a rash from touching or eating the herb. If this is the case, discontinue. If you have a clotting disorder, consult a physician before using Garlic.

In a collapse situation, it stands to reason that we may find ourselves without pharmaceutical medications. Pharmaceutical manufacture is a complex process involving a lot of chemicals (just see Dr. Bones articles on how to make Penicillin or the formula for Insulin if you don't believe me). Therefore, certain medical issues, which had relied upon these drugs, will require some form of natural treatment.

Garlic is an amazing natural medicine. It is known to be antibacterial, anti-fungal, and an immune stimulant. Garlic remedies (at least the best ones) use fresh crushed organic cloves. Used in a tea or mixed with raw, unprocessed honey, garlic has been associated with lowering blood pressure and cholesterol, and even regulating blood sugar levels.

Bacteria exposed to garlic remedies have been proven NOT to produce resistant "super-bug" strains. Antibiotic resistant organisms are becoming more and more prevalent, due to big agri-business indiscriminately using over 80% of antibiotics used today. For new or mild infections, it may be a better choice to try a natural remedy.

Garlic is versatile: For internal bacterial or fungal infections, or for respiratory congestion (to decrease tissue inflammation) use a garlic tea, or a honey garlic syrup.

For prevention or treatment of external wound infections, use: cool compresses of garlic tea (without the lemon juice); or honey garlic syrup or garlic oil, in place of a triple antibiotic ointment. Cover the wound or laceration with sterile gauze or dressing, after applying the syrup or oil. Change the covering and reapply the garlic syrup or oil once or twice daily.

Vaginal yeast infections may be cured by using a single peeled clove of garlic wrapped in a gauze and placed inside of the vagina for 8-12 hours. Remove the gauze and garlic, then place a new gauze wrapped garlic. Repeat this for 2 days. Vaginal itching can be treated with either a moist cool compress with lavender and/or tea tree essential oil added, or by sitting in a shallow warm bath of water with a few drops of the same essential oils for 15 minutes.

GARLIC What is it?

Garlic is an herb. It is best known as a flavoring for food. But over the years, garlic has been used as a medicine to prevent or treat a wide range of diseases and conditions. The fresh clove or supplements made from the clove are used for medicine.

Garlic is used for many conditions related to the heart and blood system. These conditions include high blood pressure, high cholesterol, coronary heart disease, heart attack, and "hardening of the arteries" (atherosclerosis). Some of these uses are supported by science. Garlic actually may be effective in slowing the development of atherosclerosis and seems to be able to modestly reduce blood pressure.

Some people use garlic to prevent colon cancer, rectal cancer, stomach cancer, breast cancer, prostate cancer, and lung cancer. It is also used to treat prostate cancer and bladder cancer.

Garlic has been tried for treating an enlarged prostate (benign prostatic hyperplasia; BPH), diabetes, osteoarthritis, hayfever (allergic rhinitis), traveler's diarrhea, high blood pressure late in pregnancy (pre-eclampsia), cold and flu. It is also used for building the immune system, preventing tick bites, and preventing and treating bacterial and fungal infections.

Other uses include treatment of fever, coughs, headache, stomach ache, sinus congestion, gout, rheumatism, hemorrhoids, asthma, bronchitis, shortness of breath, low blood pressure, low blood sugar, high blood sugar, and snakebites. It is also used for fighting stress and fatigue, and maintaining healthy liver function.

Some people apply garlic oil to their skin to treat fungal infections, warts, and corns. There is some evidence supporting the topical use of garlic for fungal infections like ringworm, jock itch, and athlete's foot; but the effectiveness of garlic against warts and corns is still uncertain.

There is a lot of variation among garlic products sold for medicinal purposes. The amount of allicin, the active ingredient and the source of garlic's distinctive odor, depends on the method of preparation. Allicin is unstable, and changes into a different chemical rather quickly. Some manufacturers take advantage of this by aging garlic to make it odorless. Unfortunately, this also reduces the amount of allicin and compromises the effectiveness of the product. Some odorless garlic preparations and products may contain very little, if any, allicin. Methods that involve crushing the fresh clove release more allicin. Some products have a coating (enteric coating) to protect them against attack by stomach acids.

While garlic is a common flavoring in food, some scientists have suggested that it might have a role as a food additive to prevent food poisoning. There is some evidence that fresh garlic, but not aged garlic, can kill certain bacteria such as E. coli, antibiotic-resistant Staphylococcus aureus, and Salmonella enteritidis in the laboratory.

A common ingredient for sautéing, garlic is a spice relative of onion, leek, chive and shallots. This is a common staple for many savory dishes. Although popular in the kitchen, the health benefits of garlic have also been recognized and taken advantage of since the ancient times, showing countless individuals the compelling reasons to increase garlic consumption.

Health Benefits of Garlic

Garlic has many well-known health benefits – the most popular being its anti-infection uses. Skin conditions caused by bacteria, virus, fungi or yeast can be treated by rubbing raw chopped garlic on the affected area.

Garlic is great for boosting the immune system, containing high levels of vitamin C and being identified as a serious anti-cancer food. Because of its high potassium content, it can aid in absorption of essential nutrients, and help avoid digestive problems and fatigue as well. Garlic can also help in lung and throat problems due to its pungent smell. Since consuming garlic can irritate the digestive tract because of its pungent smell, a signal travels to the brain to release watery fluid in the lungs to counter the pungent property, thereby helping clear the lungs out of cough and colds.

Adding more to the health benefits of garlic list, garlic's role in the prevention of cancer is perhaps one of the most notorious. Scientists believe that the exceptional anti-cancer properties may have to do with the way that garlic boosts the production of something known as hydrogen sulfide. It is the hydrogen sulfide production that researchers believe to be why garlic is so effective at preventing a wide variety of cancer including, prostate, breast, and colon cancer.

As an antioxidant, garlic can help protect against free radicals, cancer, high cholesterol, and can be used as one of the many home remedies for high blood pressure. It is said that the older the garlic gets, the more antioxidants properties it contain, and the more effectively it works.

To maximize on the health benefits of garlic, let it sit for a few minutes before cooking. Letting garlic sit helps to release the enzymes that provide more nutrients for the body. Raw garlic can be used to kill bacteria, but cooked garlic has more potency in lowering blood pressure and cholesterol levels. Optimally, crush the garlic at room temperature and allow it to sit for about 15 minutes. In addition, never cook garlic at high heat — try consuming it raw or cooked lightly. You can consume the spice both ways.

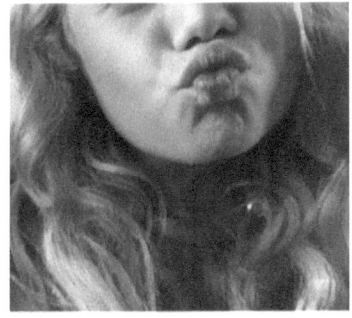 Bad breathe can be really upsetting when you are going on a date and looking for a kiss goodnight. Don't worry we have a solution to that problem. You can counter this by consuming garlic prepared as pills or capsules. If you want to get the health benefits from garlic and stave off the odor a different way, consume garlic with parsley, as the herb counters garlic's bad smell.

Not only is it antibiotic, it is also directly effective against viruses. It is also anti-fungal and anti-parasitic as well among many other things. It's important for colds AND flus.

How do I use garlic?

Well, the most obvious garlic remedy is to cook with it. I give ideas about using garlic in the immune soup recipe as well as in my special-tea. Eating garlic regularly is extremely healthful. It also helps lower blood pressure and cholesterol counts. It's absolutely amazing.

It's most potent to use garlic raw. Cooking with it regularly is good for your health, but when you need it in an acute situation, use it raw.

Juicing it and adding it to other juice is a great way to take raw.

There are many good raw garlic recipes that are garlic remedies, such as humous. This is a traditional middle eastern dish/spread. You can find it at supermarkets or you can make your own.

These recipes are a great example of "eating your medicine." Eating healthful meals with antiviral and antibiotic properties built into them is optimal. However, if you are already sick, then cooking garlic into your soup is one of your best options.

What about the odor?

If the odor is an issue or you aren't quite ready to integrate garlic into your diet more, you could try garlic tablets. Understand that tablets are never going to be as good as the real thing, but they do work.

A naturopathic doctor I know recommends this brand. They are odorless, and are well known as one of if not the best garlic tablets out there. The store I send you to on this link sell at wholesale prices. Believe me, you won't find them cheaper ANYWHERE else. The price here matches the wholesale price in my local natural foods wholesale catalog. I researched it so you don't have to.

Garlic remedy on my feet..

Two ways I use garlic when I'm sick (other than teas and soups)

Garlic vinegar. I infuse garlic in vinegar, and it's a great way to get the raw qualities of garlic. I eat the vinegar straight when I'm ill. But day-to-day, I use it in salad dressings or recipes that call for vinegar.

Garlic on my feet. Yes, you read right. Here's what I do: I crush a few garlic cloves, put them in a little jar or bowl, and cover it just so in olive oil.

In about a half hour, I rub the oil on my feet. I do this on my kids as well when they have a bad cough or they have a chest cold. For me, I also put the garlic pieces between my toes (but not for kids).

Then, I put socks on for the night and go to sleep. When I wake up, I have garlic breath, so I know it works! No kidding! Garlic enters your system and heads straight for the lungs.

Garlic is amazing for the lungs. This is a great way to fight bacterial infections. It also enhances your immune system and fights viruses at the same time! I love this garlic remedy.

Ear infections have been cured with a slice of fresh garlic clove wrapped in gauze and placed just inside of the ear. Cover the ear with a cotton ball and secure gently with a piece of paper tape. Change the garlic and gauze every 6-8 hours, until the earache is gone.Here's how to make garlic tea:

Garlic tea recipe:

1. 4 cups of filtered, boiled water, and allowed to cool slightly

2. Add 4-5 cloves of finely chopped or crushed organic garlic

3. Add fresh lemon juice and/or raw, unprocessed honey to taste

4. Drink 3-4 cups daily, either warm or cold, but do not re-boil the solution (it will stop the healing properties)

Honey Garlic Syrup recipe:

1. Crush 1/2- 1 clove garlic and place on a tablespoon

2. Pour raw, unprocessed honey onto the spoon

3. Ingest the spoonful of honey garlic syrup, every 4-6 hours, as needed Natural remedies will have to take up the slack if modern medical care and drugs are not available. Learn how to use garlic and other natural substances; you can grow them yourself, and they'll be another weapon in your medical arsenal if times get tough.

My father in law once planted a few cloves of garlic in his garden. It began to gow and he had plenty of garlic for the summer months. The following year he planted even more and was able to dry and crush the garlic bulbs as well as having fresh garlic for his soups. Try planting it and see what happens.

Yarrow

Family: Compositae Genus: Achillea Species: Millefolium

Also Known As: Bloodwort, Nose Bleed, Thousand Weed, Milfoil, Soldier's Woundwort

An excellent wound treatment, Yarrow has many healing properties, is a good digestive aid, helps menstrual cramps, and is a mild sedative.

Rx: use fresh leaves and flowers for cuts and scrapes, infusion for calming and menstrual easing effects, tincture

Warnings: large doses may turn urine brown. This is not harmful.

EATING HEALTHY

APPLES

According to a Brazilian study, eating an apple before a meal helped women lose 33 percent more weight than those who didn't. An apple has only 50-80 calories and has no fat or sodium.

Apples are packed with vitamins C, A, and flavonoids and with smaller amounts of phosphorus, iron and calcium. Apples provide a source of potassium which may promote heart health.

BERRIES

Berries are delicious, but they're also kind of delicate. Raspberries in particular seem like they can mold before you even get them home from the market. There's nothing more tragic than paying $4 for a pint of local raspberries, only to look in the fridge the next day and find that fuzzy mold growing on their insides.

Well, with fresh berries just starting to hit farmers markets, we can tell you how to prevent them from getting moldy:

Wash them with vinegar.

When you get your berries home, prepare a mixture of one part vinegar (white or apple cider) and ten parts water. Dump the berries into the mixture and swirl around. Drain, (rinse if you want, though the mixture is so diluted you can't taste the vinegar) and pop in the fridge. The vinegar kills any mold spores or other bacteria that might be on the surface of the fruit. And voila! Raspberries will last a week or more, and strawberries go almost two weeks without getting moldy and soft.

So go forth and stock up on those pricey little gems, knowing they'll stay fresh as long as it takes you to eat them.

You're so berry welcome!

Paul Davey

BRAIN FOOD

There's no denying that as we age chronologically, our body ages right along with us. But research is showing that you can increase your chances of maintaining a healthy brain well into your old age if you add these "smart" foods to your daily eating regimen.

BLUEBERRIES.

"Brainberries" is what Steven Pratt, MD, author of Superfoods Rx: Fourteen Foods Proven to Change Your Life, calls these tasty fruits. Pratt, who is also on staff at Scripps Memorial Hospital in La Jolla, Calif., says that in animal studies researchers have found that blueberries help protect the brain from oxidative stress and may reduce the effects of age-related conditions such as Alzheimer's disease or dementia. Studies have also shown that diets rich in blueberries significantly improved both the learning capacity and motor skills of aging rats, making them mentally equivalent to much younger rats. Ann Kulze, MD, author of Dr. Ann's 10-Step Diet: A Simple Plan for Permanent Weight Loss; Lifelong Vitality, recommends adding at least 1 cup of blueberries a day in any form -- fresh, frozen, or freeze-dried.

FRESHLY BREWED TEA.

Two to three cups a day of freshly brewed tea -- hot or iced -- contains a modest amount of caffeine which, when used "judiciously," says Kulze -- can boost brain power by enhancing memory, focus, and mood. Tea also has potent antioxidants, especially the class known as catechines, which promotes healthy blood flow. Bottled or powdered teas don't do the trick, however, says Kulze. "It has to be freshly brewed." Tea bags do count, however.

WILD SALMON.

Deep-water fish, such as salmon, are rich in omega-3 essential fatty acids, which are essential for brain function, says Kulze. Both she and Pratt recommend wild salmon for its "cleanliness" and the fact that it is in plentiful supply. Omega-3s also contain anti-inflammatory substances. Other oily fish that provide the benefits of omega-3s are sardines and herring, says Kulze; she recommends a 4-ounce serving, two to three times a week.

NUTS AND SEEDS.

Nuts and seeds are good sources of vitamin E, says Pratt, explaining that higher levels of vitamin E correspond with less cognitive decline as you get older. Add an ounce a day of walnuts, hazelnuts, Brazil nuts, filberts, almonds, cashews, peanuts, sunflower seeds, sesame seeds, flax seed, and unhydrogenated nut butters such as peanut butter, almond butter, and tahini. Raw or roasted doesn't matter, although if you're on a sodium-restricted diet, buy unsalted nuts.

AVOCADOS.

Avocados are almost as good as blueberries in promoting brain health, says Pratt. "I don't think the avocado gets its due," agrees Kulze. True, the avocado is a fatty fruit, but, says Kulze, it's a monounsaturated fat, which contributes to healthy blood flow. "And healthy blood flow means a healthy brain," she says. Avocados also lower blood pressure, says Pratt, and as hypertension is a risk factor for the decline in cognitive abilities, a lower blood pressure should promote brain health.

Avocados are high in calories, however, so Kulze suggests adding just 1/4 to 1/2 of an avocado to one daily meal as a side dish.

BEANS.

Beans are "under-recognized" and "economical," says Kulze. They also stabilize glucose (blood sugar) levels. The brain is dependent on glucose for fuel, Kulze explains, and since it can't store the glucose, it relies on a steady stream of energy -- which beans can provide. Any beans will do, says Kulze, but she is especially partial to lentils and black beans and recommends 1/2 cup every day.

POMEGRANATE JUICE.

Pomegranate juice (you can eat the fruit itself but with its many tiny seeds, it's not nearly as convenient) offers potent antioxidant benefits, says Kulze, which protect the brain from the damage of free radicals. "Probably no part of the body is more sensitive to the damage from free radicals as the brain," says board-certified neurologist David Perlmutter, MD, author of The Better Brain Book. Citrus fruits and colorful vegetables are also high on Perlmutter's list of "brainy" foods because of their antioxidant properties -- "the more colorful the better," he says. Because pomegranate juice has added sugar (to counteract its natural tartness), you don't want to go overboard, says Kulze; she recommends approximately 2 ounces a day, diluted with spring water or seltzer.

WHOLE GRAINS.

Whole grains, such as oatmeal, whole-grain breads, and brown rice can reduce the risk for heart disease. "Every organ in the body is dependent on blood flow," says Pratt. "If you promote cardiovascular health, you're promoting good flow to the organ system, which includes the brain." While wheat germ is not technically a whole grain, it also goes on Kulze's "superfoods" list because in addition to fiber, it has vitamin E and some omega-3s. Kulze suggests 1/2 cup of whole-grain cereal, 1 slice of bread two-thee times day, or 2 tablespoons of wheat germ a day.

DARK CHOCOLATE.

 Let's end with the good stuff. Dark chocolate has powerful antioxidant properties, contains several natural stimulants, including caffeine, which enhance focus and concentration, and stimulates the production of endorphins, which helps improve mood. One-half ounce to 1 ounce a day will provide all the benefits you need, says Kulze. This is one "superfood" where more is not better. "You have to do this one in moderation," says Kulze.

A Few Great Tips

CUCUMBERS

Health Value and Other uses..

1. Cucumbers contain most of the vitamins you need every day, just one cucumber contains Vitamin B1, Vitamin B2, Vitamin B3, Vitamin B5, Vitamin B6, Folic Acid, Vitamin C, Calcium, Iron, Magnesium, Phosphorus, Potassium and Zinc.

2. Feeling tired in the afternoon, put down the caffeinated soda and pick up a cucumber. Cucumbers are a good source of B Vitamins and carbohydrates that can provide that quick pick-me-up that can last for hours.

3. Tired of your bathroom mirror fogging up after a shower? Try rubbing a cucumber slice along the mirror, it will eliminate the fog and provide a soothing, spa-like fragrance.

4. Are grubs and slugs ruining your planting beds? Place a few slices in a small pie tin and your garden will be free of pests all season long. The chemicals in the

cucumber react with the aluminum to give off a scent undetectable to humans but drive garden pests crazy and make them flee the area.

5. Looking for a fast and easy way to remove cellulite before going out or to the pool? Try rubbing a slice or two of cucumbers along your problem area for a few minutes, the phytochemicals in the cucumber cause the collagen in your skin to tighten, firming up the outer layer and reducing the visibility of cellulite. Works great on wrinkles too!!!

6. Want to avoid a hangover or terrible headache? Eat a few cucumber slices before going to bed and wake up refreshed and headache free. Cucumbers contain enough sugar, B vitamins and electrolytes to replenish essential nutrients the body lost, keeping everything in equilibrium, avoiding both a hangover and headache!!

7. Looking to fight off that afternoon or evening snacking binge? Cucumbers have been used for centuries and often used by European trappers, traders and explorers for quick meals to thwart off starvation.

8. Have an important meeting or job interview and you realize that you don't have enough time to polish your shoes? Rub a freshly cut cucumber over the shoe, its chemicals will provide a quick and durable shine that not only looks great but also repels water.

9. Out of WD40 and need to fix a squeaky hinge? Take a cucumber slice and rub it along the problematic hinge, and voila, the squeak is gone!

10. Stressed out and don't have time for massage, facial or visit to the spa? Cut up an entire cucumber and place it in a boiling pot of water, the chemicals and nutrients from the cucumber will react with the boiling water and be released in the steam, creating a soothing, relaxing aroma that has been shown to reduce stress in new mothers and college students during final exams.

11. Just finish a business lunch and realize you don't have gum or mints? Take a slice of cucumber and press it to the roof of your mouth with your tongue for 30 seconds to eliminate bad breath, the phytochemcials will kill the bacteria in your mouth responsible for causing bad breath.

12. Looking for a 'green' way to clean your faucets, sinks or stainless steel? Take a slice of cucumber and rub it on the surface you want to clean, not only will it remove years of tarnish and bring back the shine, but it won't leave streaks and won't harm your fingers or fingernails while you clean.

13. Using a pen and made a mistake? Take the outside of the cucumber and slowly use it to erase the pen writing, also works great on crayons and markers that the kids have used to decorate the walls!!

CLEAN YOUR KIDNEYS FOR A $1.00 OR EVEN LESS

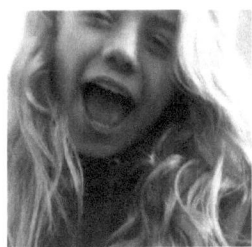

Years pass by and our kidneys are filtering the blood by removing salt, poison and any unwanted entering our body. With time, the salt accumulates and this needs to undergo cleaning treatments and how are we going to overcome this?

It is very easy, first take a bunch of parsley or Cilantro (Coriander Leaves) and wash it clean

Then cut it in small pieces and put it in a pot and pour clean water and boil it for ten minutes and let it cool down and then filter it and pour in a clean bottle and keep it inside refrigerator to cool.

Drink one glass daily and you will notice all salt and other accumulated poison coming out of your kidney by urination also you will be able to notice the difference which you never felt before.

Parsley (Cilantro) is known as best cleaning treatment for kidneys and it is natural!

COFFEE / CAFFEINE

Coffee may be the most popular drink in the world. It contains a substance called caffeine. Caffeine can be naturally found not only in coffee but tea and chocolate.

Medical practitioners usually add caffeine into pain relievers, migraine healers, etc. Caffeine is generally harmless but in some people, it has negative effects such as headaches, stomach upset, and jitters. For people with pre-existing kidney problems, coffee can also affect kidney function.

Here are the effects of coffee (or caffeine) on kidney function:

▶ Urinate more often. It is caused by diuretics effect of caffeine.

▶ Dehydration. Since coffee has diuretic effects, you have to make sure that your fluid intake is enough to prevent dehydration. Dehydration is harmful for the kidney because it can cause acute injury and promote infection on the kidney and also urinary system.

▶ Urinary incontinence. Coffee can increase the risk of urinary incontinence, especially if you drink more than 400 mg of caffeine a day.

▶ Kidney stones. Caffeine can increase urinary calcium levels. In a research, it was concluded that there was a moderate increase in the risk of developing kidney stones (especially calcium oxalate stones, the most common type of stones) after a significant caffeine consumption.

▶ Kidney disease. In a study, it is concluded that people with polycystic kidney disease were more likely to develop larger cysts if they consume caffeine because caffeine can damage kidney function.

Cravings have nothing to do with willpower!

An enormous percentage of women crave sugar, carbohydrates, or alcohol. In most cases, these food cravings are not true eating disorders, but instead are signs of hormonal imbalance caused by a lack of healthy nutrition.

Your personal issue may be the afternoon snack (often chocolate or candy or a food that's also heavy in carbohydrates), too many potato chips, the extra glass of wine at night, or a hundred other variations. But the underlying mechanism, and the way to curb cravings, is the same. And it has nothing to do with willpower, or your lack thereof!

Food cravings mean that the body has its signals mixed up. When we are exhausted or blue, we have low blood sugar and/or low serotonin, and the body signals the brain that it needs a pick-me-up. This signal causes a sugar craving or carbohydrate craving.

Serotonin is our basic feel-good hormone. If serotonin is low, we feel sad or depressed. And hormonal imbalance or weak digestion can lead to low serotonin. Unfortunately, sugars and simple carbohydrates release a short burst of serotonin — we feel good for a moment, but soon return to our low-serotonin state — then crave more sugar and simple carbohydrates. It's a downward spiral.

If you eat a low-fat diet in the hope of losing weight, you unintentionally make the problem worse. If, like millions of women, you have eaten a low-fat, high-carbohydrate diet for many years, or followed fad diets, the odds are good that you have become at least partially insulin resistant.

Insulin is responsible for maintaining stable blood sugar levels by telling the body's cells when to absorb glucose from the bloodstream. Being insulin resistant means your body stops responding to insulin, and instead grabs every calorie it can and deposits it as fat. So no matter how little you eat, you will gradually gain weight.

At the same time, your cells cannot absorb the glucose they need, so they signal your brain that you need more carbohydrates or sugars. The result is persistent food cravings.

Even worse, insulin resistance leads directly to obesity, diabetes, and heart disease. Many experts believe it is the root cause of the epidemic of those diseases in

America today. And a low-fat diet makes it far more likely you will suffer from this condition.

Millions of American women are now trying the Atkins Diet or the South Beach Diet. While these diets are an improvement over the conventional low-fat, high-carbohydrate diet, they can worsen your metabolic problems, because dieting itself is stressful to the body. So many women need to heal their metabolism first before even considering weight loss.

Another cause of food cravings is adrenal imbalance. If you are under a great deal of stress, or suffer from insomnia or sleep deprivation, you are probably exhausted much of the time. This situation causes your body to call upon your adrenal glands for more stress hormones to act as a pick-me-up, but over time, your adrenals become less able to respond appropriately. You may resort to sugar or carbohydrate snacks or coffee during the day and carbohydrates or alcohol at night, all of which exacerbate the problem.

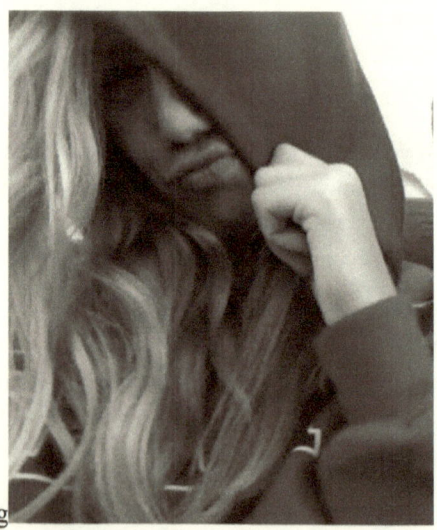

How to curb craving

Women who blame themselves for their food cravings only worsen their mood and increase their need for serotonin. That's when a pattern of emotional eating can develop. Remember, there are biological causes of sugar cravings, and your carbohydrate craving is rarely just a behavioral problem. The root problem is more likely inadequate nutrition.

How to break this vicious cycle? To reduce food cravings, the body needs real support — and lots of it. We have seen over and over that eating healthy foods, adding pharmaceutical–grade nutritional supplements and moderate exercise can almost miraculously curb cravings. Your metabolism will heal itself when provided with the necessary nutritional support. If it has been damaged, the process can take some time, but it will happen. The good news is — you don't have to give up chocolate

DETOXING THE BODY

Epsom Salts Bath

Bathing in an Epsom salts (magnesium sulphate) bath is a pleasant way to cleanse. Magnesium is absorbed through the skin which actually helps to draw toxins and heavy metals from cells, soothes and relaxes muscles, reduces swelling and has a calming effect.

Epson Salts that is taken internally acts as a detoxifying agent for colon cleansing. Drinking 1 tablespoon of Epsom salts mixed in one litre of water on an empty stomach in the morning will aid in a swift cleansing of the colon. Make sure you only do this when you know you don't have to go anywhere for the next hour.

Epsom Salts cost very little but be aware of the super cheap types. Some Epsom Salts can contain chemicals you don't want to have in your body. Epsom Salts that are advertised as 95 -100% pure are usually quite safe. Be generous with how much you place in your warm bath. Add two to four cups of the salts to running water, dim the lights, play soft music and light up a candle to give yourself a treat of relaxation whilst detoxing. Soak for at least 20 minutes. Do not use soap as it will interfere with the action of the salts. You will not need to clean with soap as Epsom salts is a wonderful cleanser for the skin, in fact Epsom salts is one of my favourite facial cleansers and a natural body scrub.

HONEY

1) HEART DISEASES: Apply honey and cinnamon powder on bread instead of using jam or butter and eat it regularly for breakfast.

2) ARTHRITIS: Apply a paste made of the two ingredients on the affected part of the body and massage slowly.

3) HAIR LOSS: Apply a paste of hot olive oil, a tablespoon of honey, a teaspoon of cinnamon powder before bath, leave it for 15 min and wash.

4) BLADDER INFECTIONS: Mix cinnamon powder and honey in a glass of lukewarm water and drink.

5) TOOTHACHE: Apply a paste of cinnamon powder and honey and on the aching tooth.

6) CHOLESTEROL: Add honey to cinnamon powder mixed in boiled water or green tea and drink.

7) COLDS: Make a glass of lukewarm honey water mixed with cinnamon powder to help boost your immune system during the cold season. It may also help to clear your sinuses.

8) INDIGESTION: Cinnamon powder sprinkled on a spoonful of honey taken before food relieves acidity.

9) LONGEVITY: Regularly take tea made with honey and a little cinnamon powder.

10) PIMPLES: Mix honey with cinnamon powder and apply paste on the pimples before sleeping and wash away the next morning.

11) OBESITY: To reduce weight, daily drink a mixture of a teaspoon of honey with half a teaspoon of cinnamon powder boiled in water with an empty stomach in the morning about half an hour before breakfast. Read: Cinnamon and Honey Recipe. <-- Don't Miss It!

Cinnamon has an insulin boosting property (water soluble compounds called polyphenol type A polymers) which have the ability to boost insulin activity about 20 fold and can benefit people who have high sugar levels (obese people, pre-diabetics and diabetics). Also, read the honey hibernation diet theory to find out how honey contributes to the metabolizing of undesirable cholesterol and fatty acid, provides a fuelling mechanism for the body, keep blood sugar levels balanced, and let our recovery hormones get on with burning body fat stores.

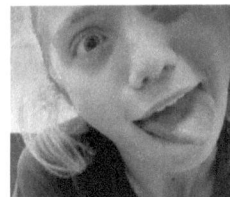 No one likes bad breath, well here is a tip that will help. I know you probably think some of this is ridiculous but it works.

The choice is yours, but I know others will be thankful that they don't have to smell your bad breathe anymore.

12) BAD BREATH: Gargle with honey and cinnamon powder mixed in hot water so that breath stays fresh throughout the day.

Honey and Cinnamon to Cure Colds

Did you know that a teaspoon of honey (local - raw is best) and a 1/4 teaspoon of cinnamon will usually knock out a cold within a day or two? Take twice a day for 3 days for best results. Both honey and cinnamon are antiviral, antibacterial, and antifungal. Also knocks bladder/kidney infections, reduces sugar levels, blood pressure and acts as a pain reliever for arthritis!

Ginger Detox Bath

Another alternative to a detox bath is to add 1/8 cup of freshly grated ginger to your bath. Ginger is wonderful for detoxing the body, opening the pores of your skin and eliminating toxins.

To enhance the effectiveness of an Epsom salts or ginger detox, make sure you drink 2 glasses of water before and after the bath. You can also gain added benefit by wrapping yourself in a towel after rubbing yourself vigorously and while you are still warm put yourself under the bed covers and try to fall asleep. You will continue to sweat for a good hour or so afterwards which will further release toxins.

HYDROGEN PEROXIDE

Hydrogen peroxide is the only germicidal agent composed only of water and oxygen. Like ozone, it kills disease organisms by oxidation! Hydrogen peroxide is considered the worlds safest all natural effective sanitizer. It kills microorganisms by oxidizing them, which can be best described as a controlled burning process. When hydrogen peroxide reacts with organic material it breaks down into oxygen and water.

1. Whiten Clothes – An Alternative to Beach

Add a cup of Peroxide to white clothes in your laundry to whiten them. Peroxide is great to get rid of blood stains on clothes and carpets. If there is blood on clothing, just pour directly on the spot, let it sit for about a minute, then rub and rinse with cold water. Repeat if necessary.

2. Health

Your body makes hydrogen peroxide to fight infection which must be present for our immune system to function correctly. White blood cells are known as Leukocytes. A sub-class of Leukocytes called Neutrophils produce hydrogen peroxide as the first line of defense against toxins, parasites, bacteria, viruses and yeast.

3. Rejuvenating Detoxifying Bath

Use about 2 quarts 3% hydrogen peroxide to a tub of warm water. Soak at least 1/2 hour, adding hot water as needed to maintain a comfortable water temperature.

4. Foot Fungus

To cure a foot fungus, simply spray a 50/50 mixture of hydrogen peroxide and water on them (especially the toes) every night and let dry.

5. Douche

Add 2 capfuls of 3% hydrogen peroxide in warm distilled water once to twice a week to remove even chronic yeast infections.

6. Colonic or Enema

For a colonic, add 1 cup (8 ozs.) 3% H202 to 5 gallons warm water. (Do not exceed this amount) For an enema, add 1 tablespoon of 3% H202 to a quart of warm distilled water.

7. Infections

Soak any infections or cuts in 3% for five to ten minutes several times a day. Even gangrene that would not heal with any medicine has been healed by soaking in hydrogen peroxide. Put half a bottle of hydrogen peroxide in your bath to help rid boils, fungus or other skin infections.

8. Bird Mites Infections

Patients infected by tiny mites report that hydrogen peroxide effectively kills the mites on their skins. They spray it on their skin a couple of times (with a few minutes in between the applications) with amazing results.

9. Sinus Infections

A tablespoon of 3% hydrogen peroxide added to 1 cup of non-chlorinated water can be used as a nasal spray. Depending on the degree of sinus involvement, one will have to adjust the amount of peroxide used.

10. Wound Care

3% H2O2 is used medically for cleaning wounds, removing dead tissue, and as an oral debriding agent. Peroxide stops slow (small vessel) wound bleeding/oozing, as well.

Some sources recommend soaking infections or cuts for five to ten minutes several times a day. However, washing and rinsing action is sufficient. You shouldn't leave the solution on open tissue for extended periods of time as, like many oxidative antiseptics, hydrogen perioxide causes mild damage to tissue in open wounds. Therefore it is important to use with caution.

Hydrogen Peroxide

Mouthwash / Tooth Care

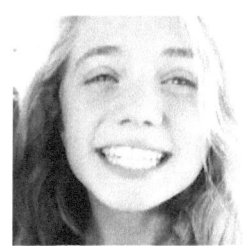

Healing Properties: Take one capful (the little white cap that comes with the bottle) and hold in your mouth for 10 minutes daily, then spit it out. You will not have canker sores and your teeth will be whiter. If you have a terrible toothache and cannot get to a dentist right away, put a capful of 3% hydrogen peroxide into your mouth and hold it for 10 minutes several times a day. The pain will lessen greatly.

11. Mouthwash

Many people don't realize that hydrogen peroxide makes a very effective and inexpensive mouthwash. Use 3% H202 – add a dash of liquid chlorophyll for flavoring if desired.

12. Toothpaste

Use baking soda and add enough 3% H202 to make a paste.

13. Toothbrush

Or, just dip your brush in 3% H202 and brush. Soak your toothbrush in hydrogen peroxide to keep them free of germs.

14. Tooth Ache

Hydrogen peroxide is not a pain killer; however, as an anti-viral, antibacterial and anti-fungal agent, it is effective at treating the pathogen that is causing the infection. The following is from my own personal experience: My dentist wanted to give me a root canal some time ago as one tooth was inflamed and, in her opinion, would die. I felt some discomfort but told her that I would give it chance to heal. I rinsed with hydrogen peroxide (several times a day) as well ascoconut oil (once a day). The discomfort went away and I have had no further problems with the tooth.

15. Tooth Whitening

Having used 3% Hydrogen Peroxide as a mouth wash for sometime ago, I am thrilled to note that my teeth have been beautifully and effortlessly whitened. I used to pay so much for professional whitening, those silly strips and uncomfortable trays. Live and learn.

NOTE: Do not swallow any peroxide. When the peroxide rinse is done, be sure to rinse out your mouth with water.

16. Hair Lightening

Peroxide is a bleaching agent and is used for lightened hair. Dilute 3% hydrogen peroxide with water (50 / 50) and spray the solution on your wet hair after a shower and comb it through. You will not have the peroxide burnt blonde hair like the hair dye packages, but more natural highlights if your hair is a light brown, faddish, or dirty blonde. It also lightens gradually so it's not a drastic change.

17. Contact Lenses

Hydrogen peroxide is used as a disinfectant in CIBA Vision's Clear Care no rub contact lens cleaning solution, due to its ability to break down the proteins that build up on the lense from the eye's immune response, resulting in increased comfort for those with sensitive eyes.

Sanitizing / Disinfectant / Cleaning

18. Straight or Diluted Hydrogen Perioxide

Clean your counters and table tops with hydrogen peroxide to kill germs and leave a fresh smell. Simply put a little on your dishrag when you wipe, or spray it on the counters. Use hydrogen peroxide to clean glass and mirrors with no smearing.

Keep a spray bottle of 3% (straight) to disinfect the interior of the refrigerator and kids' school lunch boxes.

19. In the Dishwasher

Add 2 oz. of 3% hydrogen peroxide to your regular washing formula.

Fill a spray bottle with a 50/50 mixture of 3% hydrogen peroxide and water and keep it in every bathroom to disinfect without harming your septic system like bleach or most other disinfectants will. After rinsing off your wooden cutting board, pour or spray hydrogen peroxide (and then vinegar) on it to kill salmonella and other bacteria.

I use peroxide to clean my mirrors with, there is no smearing.

Combination of vinegar and hydrogen peroxidemake a cheap, effective and non-toxic disinfectant agent and is said to be more effective at killing pathogens than bleach. As it is non-toxic, you can use it to disinfect fruits and vegetables, as well as pet toys, equipment and cages. In tests run at Virginia Polytechnic Institute and State University, pairing Vinegar and Hydrogen Peroxide mists, kills virtually all Salmonella, Shigella, or E. coli bacteria on heavily contaminated food and surfaces.

Directions

You need TWO spray bottles. DO NOT MIX the solutions together. Put straight vinegar in one and straight hydrogen peroxide in the other spray bottle.

NOTE: Light destroys peroxide rather quickly. It's best to leave it in its original bottle and screw in a spray head. DO NOT DILUTE THEM.

Remember for any sanitizer to work properly, the surface has to be clean before you use it.

When you want to sanitize a surface (vegetables, cutting board, counters, sink, cages, toys. toilets, floors, etc.), spray one (it doesn't matter which one you use first) on the surface, then you spray on the other. When they mix, for a brief time the chemical action of the two make a very powerful sanitizer. You can rinse off the surface afterwards, if you want, but the result is non-toxic.

Fortunately it is cheap. BTW, we use it in the bathroom to sanitize the counters, toilets, floors, etc.

20. Mold

Clean with hydrogen peroxide when your house becomes a biohazard after its invaded by toxic mold, such as those with water damage.

21. Humidifiers/Steamers

Use 1 pint 3% hydrogen peroxide to 1 gallon of water.

22. Laundry / Stain Removing

Stain Remover

3% Hydrogen Peroxide is the best stain lifter if used fairly soon – although blood stains as old as 2 days have been successfully lifted with Hydrogen Peroxide. Although it will bleach or discolor many fabrics. If a little peroxide is poured onto the stain it will bubble up in the area of the blood, due to a reaction with catalase. After a few minutes the excess liquid can be wiped up with a cloth or paper towel and the stain will be gone.

3% H2O2 must be applied to clothing before blood stains can be accidentally "set" with heated water. Cold water and soap are then used to remove the peroxide treated blood.

23. Washing/Laundry

You can also add a cup of hydrogen peroxide instead of bleach to a load of whites in your laundry to whiten them. If there is blood on clothing, pour directly on the soiled spot. Let it sit for a minute, then rub it and rinse with cold water. Repeat if necessary.

Peroxide is a perfect alternate solution to keep those clothes white. Also, when chlorinating clothes, they tend to wear out faster – peroxide won't do that.

Food Preparation

24. Vegetable Soak

Use as a vegetable wash or soak to kill bacteria and neutralize chemicals. Add 1/4 cup 3% H202 to a full sink of cold water. Soak light skinned (light lettuce) 20 minutes, thicker skinned (like cucumbers) 30 minutes. Drain, dry and refrigerate. Prolongs freshness.

If time is a problem, spray vegetables (and fruits) with a solution of 3%. Let stand for a few minutes, rinse and dry.

25. Meat Sanitizing

You can also use it to rinse off your meat before cooking.

26. Leftover tossed salad

Spray with a solution of 1/2 cup water and 1 Tbsp. 5%. Drain, cover and refrigerate.

27. Marinade

Place meat, fish or poultry in a casserole (avoid using aluminium pans). Cover with a dilute solution of equal parts of water and 3% H202. Place loosely covered in refrigerator for 1/2 hour. Rinse and cook.

28. Sprouting Seeds

Add 1 ounce 3% hydrogen peroxide to 1 pint of water and soak the seeds overnight. Add the same amount of hydrogen peroxide each time you rinse the seeds.

Grades of Hydrogen Peroxide

A) 3.5% Pharmaceutical Grade: This is the grade sold at your local drugstore or supermarket. This product is not recommended for internal use. It contains an assortment of stabilizers which shouldn't be ingested. Various stabilizers include: acetanilide, phenol, sodium stanate and tertrasodium phosphate.

B) 6% Beautician Grade: This is used in beauty shops to color hair and is not recommended for internal use.

C) 30% Reagent Grade: This is used for various scientific experimentation and also contains stabilizers. It is also not for internal use.

Useful info

DID YOU know that you can treat your illness using safe and effective natural home remedies? Try the following simple remedies as advised by experts:

1. Make MUSCLE PAIN a memory with GINGER

When Danish researchers asked achy people to jazz up their diets with ginger, it eased muscle and joint pain, swelling and stiffness for up to 63 percent of them within two months. Experts credit ginger's potent compounds called gingerols, which prevent the production of pain-triggering hormones. The study-recommended dose: Add at least 1 teaspoon of dried ginger or 2 teaspoons of chopped ginger to meals daily.

2. Cure a TOOTHACHE with CLOVES

Got a toothache and can't get to the dentist? Gently chewing on a clove can ease tooth pain and gum inflammation for two hours straight, say UCLA researchers. Experts point to a natural compound in cloves called eugenol, a powerful, natural anesthetic. Bonus: Sprinkling a ¼ teaspoon of ground cloves on meals daily may also protect your ticker. Scientists say this simple action helps stabilize blood sugar, plus dampen production of artery-clogging cholesterol in as little as three weeks.

3. Heal HEARTBURN with CIDER VINEGAR

Sip 1 tablespoon of apple cider vinegar mixed with 8 ounces of water before every meal, and experts say you could shut down painful bouts of heartburn in as little as 24 hours. "Cider vinegar is rich in malic and tartaric acids, powerful digestive aids that speed the breakdown of fats and proteins so your stomach can empty quickly, before food washes up into the esophagus, triggering heartburn pain," explains Joseph Brasco, M.D., a gastroenterologist at the Center for Colon and Digestive Diseases in Huntsville, AL.

4. Erase EARACHES with GARLIC

Painful ear infections drive millions of Americans to doctors' offices every year. To cure one fast, just place two drops of warm garlic oil into your aching ear twice daily for five days. This simple treatment can clear up ear infections faster than prescription meds, say experts at the University of New Mexico School of Medicine. Scientists say garlic's active ingredients (germanium, selenium, and sulfur compounds) are naturally toxic to dozens of different pain-causing bacteria. To whip up your own garlic oil gently simmer three cloves of crushed garlic in a half a cup of extra virgin olive oil for two minutes, strain, then refrigerate for up to two weeks, suggests Teresa Graedon, Ph.D., co-author of the book, Best Choices

From The People's Pharmacy . For an optimal experience, warm this mix slightly before using so the liquid will feel soothing in your ear canal.

5. Chase away JOINT and HEADACHE PAIN with CHERRIES

Latest studies show that at least one in four women is struggling with arthritis, gout or chronic headaches. If you're one of them, a daily bowl of cherries could ease your ache, without the stomach upset so often triggered by today's painkillers, say researchers at East Lansing's Michigan State University. Their research reveals that anthocyanins, the compounds that give cherries their brilliant red color, are anti-inflammatories 10 times stronger than ibuprofen and aspirin. "Anthocyanins help shut down the powerful enzymes that kick-start tissue inflammation, so they can prevent, as well as treat, many different kinds of pain," explains Muraleedharan Nair, Ph.D., professor of food science at Michigan State University. His advice: Enjoy 20 cherries (fresh, frozen or dried) daily, then continue until your pain disappears.

6. FIGHT TUMMY TROUBLES with FISH

Indigestion, irritable bowel syndrome, inflammatory bowel diseases...if your belly always seems to be in an uproar, try munching 18 ounces of fish weekly to ease your misery. Repeated studies show that the fatty acids in fish, called EPA and DHA, can significantly reduce intestinal inflammation, cramping and belly pain and, in some cases, provide as much relief as corticosteroids and other prescription meds. "EPA and DHA are powerful, natural, side effect-free anti-inflammatories, that can dramatically improve the function of the entire gastrointestinal tract," explains biological chemist Barry Sears, Ph.D., president of the Inflammation Research Foundation in Marblehead, MA. For best results, look for oily fish like salmon, sardines, tuna, mackerel, trout and herring.

7. Prevent PMS with YOGURT

Up to 80 percent of women will struggle with premenstrual syndrome and its uncomfortable symptoms, report Yale researchers. The reason: Their nervous systems are sensitive to the ups and downs in estrogen and progesterone that occur naturally every month. But snacking on 2 cups of yogurt a day can slash these symptoms by 48 percent, say researchers at New York's Columbia University. "Yogurt is rich in calcium, a mineral that naturally calms the nervous system, preventing painful symptoms even when hormones are in flux," explains Mary Jane Minkin, M.D., a professor of gynecology at Yale University.

8. TAME CHRONIC PAIN with TURMERIC

Studies show turmeric, a popular East Indian spice, is actually three times more effective at easing pain than aspirin, ibuprofen or naproxen, plus it can help relieve chronic pain for 50 percent of people struggling with arthritis and even fibromyalgia, according to Cornell researchers. That's because turmeric's active ingredient, curcumin, naturally shuts down cyclooxygenase 2, an enzyme that churns out a stream of pain-producing hormones, explains nutrition researcher Julian Whitaker, M.D. and author of the book, REVERSING DIABETES. The study-recommended dose: Sprinkle 1/4 teaspoon of this spice daily onto any rice, poultry, meat or vegetable dish.

9. OATS for FAST PAIN RELIEF

It's not for Breakfast anymore!..

Mix 2 cups of OATS and 1 cup of water in a bowl and warm in Microwave for 1 minute, cool slightly,

and APPLY the mixture to your hands for soothing relief from ARTHRITIS PAIN.

10. Soothe FOOT PAIN WITH SALT

Experts say at least six million Americans develop painful ingrown toenails each year. But regularly soaking ingrown nails in warm salt water baths can cure these painful infections within four days, say scientists at California's Stanford University. The salt in the mix naturally nixes inflammation, plus it's anti-bacterial, so it quickly destroys the germs that cause swelling and pain. Just mix 1 teaspoon of salt into each cup of water, heat to the warmest temperature that you can comfortably stand, and then soak the affected foot area for 20 minutes twice daily, until your infection subsides.

11. PREVENT DIGESTIVE UPSETS with PINEAPPLE

Got gas? One cup of fresh pineapple daily can cut painful bloating within 72 hours, say researchers at California's Stanford University. That's because pineapple is naturally packed with proteolytic enzymes, digestive aids that help speed the breakdown of pain-causing proteins in the stomach and small intestine, say USDA researchers.

12. RELAX PAINFUL MUSCLES with PEPPERMINT

Suffering from tight, sore muscles? Stubborn knots can hang around for months if they aren't properly treated, says naturopath Mark Stengler, N.D., author of the book, The Natural Physician's Healing Therapies . His advice: Three times each week, soak in a warm tub scented with 10 drops of peppermint oil. The warm water will relax your muscles, while the peppermint oil will naturally soothe your nerves -- a combo that can ease muscle cramping 25 percent more effectively than over-the-counter painkillers, and cut the frequency of future flare-ups in half, says Stengler.

10 Health Benefits of Chocolate

1. High in Antioxidants

Cocoa contains flavanols, a type of flavanoid that is only found in cocoa and chocolate. Flavanoids are naturally-occurring compounds that occur in plant foods that act as antioxidants and help counteract free radicals in the body.

2. Blood Pressure Benefits

Dark chocolate has been shown in studies to lower blood pressure in people with elevated blood pressure.

3. Lower LDL Cholesterol

Eating dark chocolate on a regular basis has been shown to reduce LDL cholesterol by as much as 10 percent.

4. Natural Anti-Depressant

Chocolate contains serotonin, a natural anti-depressant. Chocolate also stimulates endorphin production, which creates feelings of happiness and pleasure. In fact, one study found that melting chocolate in the mouth produced feelings of pleasure longer than passionate kissing. This may explain why many people naturally reach for chocolate when they're depressed.

5. Cancer Fighter

Several studies have found chocolate to be one of the best cancer-fighting foods along with foods like red wine, blueberries, garlic, and tea. Two ways that chocolate works as a cancer fighter is by inhibiting cell division and reducing inflammation, though research is ongoing and will probably find additional ways in which chocolate fights cancer.

6. Prevents Tooth Decay

Research has found that the theobromine in chocolate prevents tooth decay by eliminating streptococcus mutans, a bacteria found in the oral cavity that contributes to tooth decay.

7. Longer Life and Less Disease

One Dutch study followed 200 men over 20 years and found that those who consumed large amounts of chocolate, both milk chocolate and dark, lived longer and had lower overall disease rates than men who ate little or no chocolate.

A Harvard study on the Kuna tribe of Panama resulted in similar findings. The Kuna consumed large amounts of raw cacao every day and the study found them to have lower overall disease rates and longer life expectancy than neighboring tribes who did not consume as much raw cacao.

To further strengthen the case for dark chocolate as a life extender, the world's longest-lived person, Jeanne Louise Calment, lived to the age of 122 and many ascribed her longevity in part to her consumption of 2.5 pounds of dark chocolate a week.

8. High in Magnesium

Cacao is higher in magnesium than any other plant. Magnesium is an important mineral that helps in the regulation of the digestive, neurological, and cardiovascular systems. Since many people are magnesium deficient, adding magnesium-rich dark chocolate to the diet can improve overall health.

9. Artery Cleanup

Studies have shown that the antioxidants in cacao work like brooms in sweeping plaque out of the arteries.

10. Brain Health

Many studies have shown that dark chocolate is good for the brain. Researchers at Johns Hopkins University found it can protect the brain after a stroke by shielding nerve cells from further damage. Dark chocolate has also been found to improve memory. Researchers at California's Salk found that a chemical in chocolate called epicatechin improved the memory of mice.

Useful info

ONIONS!

In 1919 when the flu killed 40 million people there was this Doctor that visited the many farmers to see if he could help them combat the flu...

Many of the farmers and their families had contracted it and many died.

The doctor came upon this one farmer and to his surprise, everyone was very healthy. When the doctor asked what the farmer was doing that was different the wife replied that she had placed an unpeeled onion in a dish in the rooms of the home, (probably only two rooms back then). The doctor couldn't believe it and asked if he could have one of the onions and place it under the microscope. She gave him one and when he did this, he did find the flu virus in the onion. It obviously absorbed the bacteria, therefore, keeping the family healthy.

Now, I heard this story from my hairdresser. She said that several years ago, many of her employees were coming down with the flu, and so were many of her customers. The next year she placed several bowls with onions around in her shop. To her surprise, none of her staff got sick. It must work. Try it and see what happens. We did it last year and we never got the flu.

Now there is a P. S. to this for I sent it to a friend in Oregon who regularly contributes material to me on health issues. She replied with this most interesting experience about onions:

Thanks for the reminder. I don't know about the farmer's story...but, I do know that I contacted pneumonia, and, needless to say, I was very ill... I came across an article that said to cut both ends off an onion put it into an empty jar, and place the jar next to the sick patient at night. It said the onion would be black in the morning from the germs...sure enough it happened just like that...the onion was a mess and I began to feel better.

Another thing I read in the article was that onions and garlic placed around the room saved many from the black plague years ago. They have powerful antibacterial, antiseptic properties.

This is the other note. Lots of times when we have stomach problems we don't know what to blame. Maybe it's the onions that are to blame. Onions absorb bacteria is the reason they are so good at preventing us from getting colds and flu and is the very reason we shouldn't eat an onion that has been sitting for a time after it has been cut open.

Onions are so good when fresh, we use them in our cooking, on our hamburgers and they just give that added bit of flavor that so many of us enjoy.

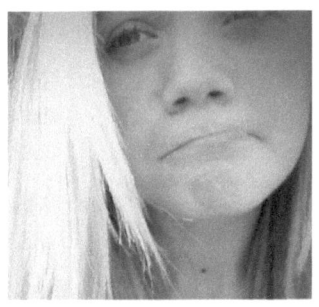

BUT, left over onions are poisonous. Yes that is what I said, Poisonous. Bet you never thought that an onion could be a poison. I sure never did. I used to put the left over onion in a plastic bag and store in the refrigerator until I needed it next. If I had only known I think it would have saved me a lot of stomach aches ..

LEFT OVER ONIONS ARE POISONOUS

 Mayonnaise is quite safe it is the onion and potatoes that attract bacteria.

When food poisoning is reported, the first thing the officials look for is when the 'victim' last ate ONIONS and where those onions came from (in the potato salad?). Ed says it's not the mayonnaise (as long as it's not homemade mayo) that spoils in the outdoors. It's probably the ONIONS, and if not the onions, it's the POTATOES.

Onions are a huge magnet for bacteria, especially uncooked onions. You should never plan to keep a portion of a sliced onion..It's not even safe if you put it in a zip-lock bag and put it in your refrigerator.

It's already contaminated enough just by being cut open and out for a bit, that it can be a danger to you. If you take the leftover onion and cook it like crazy you'll probably be okay, but if you slice that leftover onion and put on your sandwich, you're asking for trouble. Both the onions and the moist potato in a potato salad, will attract and grow bacteria faster than any commercial mayonnaise will even begin to break down.

Also, dogs should never eat onions. Their stomachs cannot metabolize onions.

Please remember it is dangerous to cut an onion and try to use it to cook the next day, it becomes highly poisonous for even a single night and creates toxic bacteria which may cause adverse stomach infections because of excess bile secretions and even food poisoning.

WAIT, don't go away I have some good news about Onions

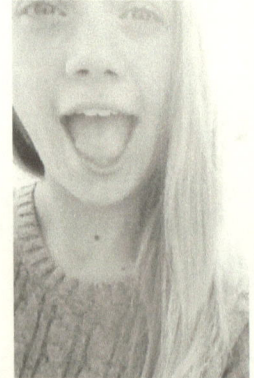

In 1919 when the flu killed 40 million people there was this Doctor that visited the many farmers to see if he could help them combat the flu...

Many of the farmers and their families had contracted it and many died.

The doctor came upon this one farmer and to his surprise, everyone was very healthy. When the doctor asked what the farmer was doing that was different

the wife replied that she had placed an unpeeled onion in a dish in the rooms of the home, (probably only two rooms back then). The doctor couldn't believe it and asked if he could have one of the onions and place it under the microscope. She gave him one and when he did this, he did find the flu virus in the onion. It obviously absorbed the bacteria, therefore, keeping the family healthy.

Now, I heard this story from my friend who runs a business in town, She said that several years ago, many of her employees were coming down with the flu, and so were many of her customers. The next year she placed several bowls with onions around in her shop. To her surprise, none of her staff got sick. It must work. Try it and see what happens.

I came across an article that said to cut both ends off an onion put it into an empty jar, and place the jar next to the sick patient at night. It said the onion would be black in the morning from the germs...sure enough it happened just like that...the onion was a mess and they began to feel better.

Once I was asked for lunch by the lady next door. Now this lady was about 86 years old and her companion, an old man about 96. When I went in I wanted to help with the lunch and to my surprise the table was set. In the middle of the table was a large bowl of onions. I would say probably 2 large onions cut up. I asked what the onions were for and the old gentleman said that each day at noon he ate a large bowl of raw onions with his lunch. He looked at me and told me to do the same. He said "That is why I have lived to be the grand old age of 96". I was totally amazed.

OLIVE OIL & COCONUT OIL

It is clear that olive oil has many helpful qualities. It strengthens hair, it removes makeup, it softens skin, and even makes a great furniture polish. But could it really help people lose weight?

 If a person who takes 2 teaspoons of olive oil every day, it will boost their metabolism. It does promote weight loss, but there are also a list of other benefits.

Dry and peeling winter skin is quickly repaired. In addition, it is full of antioxidants, cleanses the colon, and prevents gall stones.

An olive oil experiment was performed. In this experiment a person ate olive oil on fresh bread for several days in a row. They quickly realized they were losing weight and also in a better mood. In addition they discovered that their appetite was not what it had been, and they were turned off from sweets. They did not take olive oil every day, but instead ate it in spurts on bread as they craved it. This blogger cautions against overdoing it but points out the benefits of a Mediterranean diet which includes Olive Oil.

There is also much talk and evidence that coconut oil has a similar effect this is good news to me because I can have coconut oil when I am craving sweet, and olive oil when I am craving savory. After reading about other benefits like relieving joint issues and improving mood and hair (Use Coconut Oil to Grow Your African American Hair).

Everyone knows that olive oil is good for you. It has been ingrained in our brains. Extra virgin olive oil is the best. But did you know that once heated it loses many of its benefits? This is where coconut oil comes in. Extra virgin coconut oil (vco), is the only healthy oil that retains its nutritional qualities and benefits at very high temperatures making it the best oil to cook with.

Extra Virgin coconut oil is good for the heart, promotes weight loss by speeding up your metabolism and helping with the proper function of the thyroid gland, keeps your breath fresh, makes a wonderful skin moisturizer and softener, also works well as a sunscreen and does not wash off as easily as sunscreen lotions, works as an underarm and foot deodorant and as an antiperspirant. The benefits of coconut oil are countless!

Polyunsaturated fats and omega-6 oils which include common vegetable oils such as corn, soy, safflower, sunflower and canola, are the absolute worst oils to use in cooking. These oils are highly susceptible to heat damage due to the double bonds found in them and encourage the formation of blood clots by increasing platelet stickiness. Coconut oil helps to promote normal platelet function and that the only oil that is able to resist heat induced damage while promoting heart health and maintaining normal cholesterol levels is virgin coconut oil. Coconut oil is made from the flesh of matured coconuts and according to Wikipedia has 862 calories per 100 grams while olive oil has 890 calories per 100 grams. During world war II the U.S was prevented from shipping coconut oil and so other oils that were easy to obtain but not easy on the body were marketed and advertised as being good for you. After the war, coconut oil was available but kept in the dark because it threatened the market for the leading oil brands

So now I'm just passing the word. There's two types of oils you can have in your house and feel good about, extra virgin olive oil and extra virgin coconut oil. Uncooked extra virgin olive oil for your health, salad dressings and flavoring foods and coconut oil for cooking, baking and everything else including deep frying! You can get rid of those other oils. Let someone figure out how to use them in cars.

Just like olive oil there are different grades of coconut oil. For extra virgin coconut oil to benefit you it should have certain qualities. Virgin coconut oil must be organic, must not be refined, must not have added chemicals, must not be bleached, must not be deodorized, must not be hydrogenated, and must be made without heat processing. Extra Virgin Coconut Oil has a mild but pleasant flavor and scent making it a wonderful ingredient to add to your meals and your life.

1. Olive oil is not just for baking in bread recipes, it can be used for most baked good recipes that call for oil. You don't have to worry about having a strong olive oil taste in baked sweets and treats if you use Light olive oil. Light olive oil is perfect for baking cakes and sweet rolls and flavored breads.

2. Use olive oil in your marinade recipes for meat, fish, and poultry. The texture and flavor it adds is pleasant and healthy.

3. You can reduce fat in baking by using olive oil instead of butter A general rule is to use about 25 % less when replacing butter with olive oil. So, for example, if a cake recipe calls for 1 cup of butter, use 3/4 cup of Light Olive oil instead. If a recipe calls for 1/3 cup of butter use 1/4 cup of Light Olive oil instead.

4. Use olive oil for roasting vegetables. You can add seasonings you like and cover in foil. The vegetables are enhanced and retain their natural juices.

5. Olive oil drizzled over a whole bulb of garlic, then roasted in foil with some ground black pepper makes for a great spread over hot bread and garlic bread. You can sprinkle Parmesan cheese over the soft garlic spread for even more kick.

6. Store olive oil upright and in a cool, dark place. Although it can be refrigerated, it is better not to. Containers should be sealed tightly. It is better not to transfer the olive oil into plastic or metal jars or decanters because it transforms the oil and breaks down some of the flavor as well as its shelf life. Unused olive oil should be kept in its original jar, and olive oil you use to make salad dressings should be kept in glass jars with tightly fitting lids. Use your olive oil within a year of purchase.

7. Toss steamed vegetables with a tablespoon of olive oil and sprinkle with garlic powder and ground black pepper or crushed red pepper for great flavored vegetables.

8. Brush olive oil over grilled meat, poultry, or seafood right before serving. They will be tender and delicious.

9. Buy olive oil in the largest bottle you can afford, consistent with your usage. The olive oil in the larger bottles ages slower because there is less oxygen per ounce of liquid.

10. Olive oil heated and mixed with sun-dried tomatoes and Parmesan cheese makes an excellent simple, tasty and healthy dressing for cooked pasta.

11. Tossing cooked pasta with just a teaspoon of olive oil right after the pasta is drained, not only enhances the flavor, but it prevents pasta from clumping.

12. Extra Virgin Olive oil makes great dipping oil for hot crusty Italian bread or other hearty artisan breads. It can be used plain or you can create your own exotic flavor by blending some of your favorite spices and herbs.

13. A little olive oil added to butter in the frying pan, helps prevent the butter from burning.

14. Using olive oil with red wine vinegar or balsamic vinegar and a dash of black pepper and garlic powder makes a great salad dressing over salad greens. You can

also make a tasty and nutritious marinated cold vegetable salad, such as three-bean salad, or mushroom chickpea salad, by blending vegetables and beans with some olive oil and red vinegar and salt and black pepper.

15. Drizzle extra virgin olive oil over thinly sliced ripe tomatoes and mozzarella cheese and sprinkle with fresh basil and ground black pepper for a light and tasty Italian salad.

16. Olive oil is great for frying. It can take high temperatures and doesn't break down and form toxic compounds like other oils used for frying. As a result, olive oil can be re-used for frying up to four times if you filter it.

17. If you are sensitive to spicy foods, then adding extra virgin olive oil to food that is too spice will help make the flavor milder.

18. Extra virgin and virgin olive oil which is more expensive than just "olive oil" makes for better finishing oils - - the oil you use to drizzle over salad or pasta or bread.

19. Try using olive oil instead of butter on baked potatoes and mashed potatoes. It is healthy and makes for a silky texture.

20. Make your own Tabouli by using couscous and adding olive oil, chopped tomatoes, black pepper, lemon juice and scallions. Tabouli is a Middle Eastern salad dish eaten cold and often sold in the deli department of your grocery store or natural food store. But you can save money by making this simple dish at home.

COCONUT OIL

NaturalNews) Research indicates, animal fats have long chain saturated fat, while coconut oil contains healthy, healing, medium chain triglycerides (MCTs). This saturated fat is considered a rare and important building block of every cell in the human body, and can actually reduce cholesterol and heart disease.

This incredible food boosts immunity, kills bacteria and viruses, protects against cancer and other degenerative diseases, and prevents osteoporosis by promoting calcium absorption. It also slows down ageing and is good for skin radiance.

Weight Loss from Coconut Oil/Butter

American farmers attempted to plump up their cattle by feeding them coconut oil. Instead of gaining weight, their cows lost weight!

This is because:

1. The long-chain fats nearly always go to fat storage, while the MCFAs (medium chain fatty acids) are burned for energy... which is why you feel great after eating this coconut super food.

2. Coconut oil helps to stimulate the metabolism, so you burn more calories each day, which helps with weight loss and energy levels.

Coconut Oil/Butter is Packed with Lauric Acid

Coconut oil, like human breast milk, is rich in lauric acid, which boosts immunity and destroys harmful bacteria and viruses. In fact, coconut oil is one of the closest foods on the planet to breast milk.

Scientists in the Philippines researched the effects of coconut oil and lauric acid on patients with the HIV virus that causes Aids. The results were amazing. Most of the Aids patients showed a dramatic drop in the HIV virus count, in some cases to "undetectable" levels. While there needs to be a lot more research, there is certainly evidence to suggest that people with this virus would benefit from having a diet rich in coconut.

Lipid researcher Dr. Jon Kabara says "Never before in the history of man is it so important to emphasize the value of Lauric Oils."

Coconut Oil/Butter Kills Candida (Yeast Infections)

Coconut oil has been shown to kill the Candida Albicans yeast, which is caused by antibiotics, birth control pills, and modern living. It has caused a whole generation to be tired, foggy headed, unable to optimally digest food, and suffer from a range of other illnesses.

Yet many sufferers have claimed that their health has dramatically improved when using coconut products. This could be due to the fact that coconuts are a dense source of caprylic acid, which has anti-fungal properties. It could also be due to the fact that these people replaced regular milk (which is generally toxic and bad for candida sufferers) with the milk from coconuts.

Healthy Skin

Coconut Oil/Butter has youth enhancing, glow encouraging properties for the skin. It is highly moisturizing and promotes skin elasticity. I use Coconut Oil for so many things now. One is on my dog if she has a rash, it helps her stop itching and she will lick it and also get the benefits of it. I use it to condition my hair. I rub it into my scalp and hair and leave on for about an hour and then wash out. It makes a real good conditioner. Also, I put it on my face and hands as a moisturizer. Read on at some of the comments I found about Coconut Oil.

Natural News) My world is full of coconuts, including coconut oil and coconut milk. That's not unusual because I live on Maui. But I'm happily seeing coconut oil all over the internet as the treatment for dozens of conditions and possibly hundreds of symptoms.

My first clue as to the wonders of coconut oil came during my AIDS research in New York in the very early 1990's. Anecdotal reports started to pop up throughout the AIDS community about miraculous cures using coconut oil. To my mind, that's when the whole coconut oil industry opened up.

Before then, coconut oil was considered a "dangerous" saturated oil by the margarine promoters who set out to demonize butter. We know that ended in tears when it finally came out that the trans fats in margarine proved to be much more dangerous than any saturated fats.

My latest clue is the new book by Dr. Bruce Fife Stop Alzheimer's Now! that I just finished reading It's Dr. Fife's 9th book on the incredible benefits of coconut. Each year the research catches up with what he's known all along about the power of coconut oil and its completely non-toxic nature.

Dr. Fife's book presents a breakthrough in the treatment of Alzheimer's and other neurological diseases. The introduction by my friend Dr. Russell Blaylock is glowing with praise for Dr. Fife's work. And the body of the book gives a thorough overview of Alzheimer's and related diseases and then offers immense hope to people with these conditions.

As Dr. Fife's says on his website (www.coconutresearchcenter.org) "Coconut is highly nutritious and rich in fiber, vitamins, and minerals. It is classified as a 'functional food' because it provides many health benefits beyond its nutritional content. Coconut oil is of special interest because it possesses healing properties far beyond that of any other dietary oil and is extensively used in traditional medicine among Asian and Pacific populations. Pacific Islanders consider coconut oil to be the cure for all illness. The coconut palm is so highly valued by them as both a source of food and medicine that it is called 'The Tree of Life.' Only recently has modern medical science unlocked the secrets to coconut's amazing healing powers."

Dr. Fife says that "Nearly one third of the world's population depends on coconut to some degree for their food and their economy. Wherever the coconut palm grows the people have learned of its importance as an effective medicine. For thousands of years coconut products have held a respected and valuable place in local folk medicine."

Coconut oil differs from other oils because it's rich in medium chain fatty acids that are utilized readily by the body for energy.

Fats and oils are called fatty acids and they are saturated, monounsaturated or polyunsaturated fatty acids. They can also be classified as short-chain (SCFA), medium-chain (MCFA), and long-chain fatty acids (LCFA). Another term you will often see in reference to fatty acids is triglyceride. Three fatty acids joined together make a triglyceride, so you may have short-chain (SCT), medium-chain (MCT), or long-chain triglycerides (LCT).

Most dietary fats and oils you eat, whether they are saturated or unsaturated or are sourced from animals or plants, are composed of long-chain triglycerides. Almost 100% of all the fats we eat are LCT.

Now here's the point about coconut oil. It's mostly an MCT fat. Medium-chain triglycerides are exceptionally easy to digest and absorb. In my experience they don't make you burp like other fats! They are easily digested and are used by the body as a quick source of energy. But at the same time these fats give your stomach a feeling of fullness allowing you to eat less.

Most MCT products are made from coconut oil. Since they are added to infant formulas and health recovery products and athletic products more research is being done on their beneficial effects of late.

Dr. Fife graciously allowed me to quote from his website the current research on coconut oil that confirms the following extensive list of benefits.

Anti-infective Properties

*Kills viruses that cause influenza, herpes, measles, hepatitis C, SARS, AIDS, and other illnesses.

*Kills bacteria that cause ulcers, throat infections, urinary tract infections, gum disease and cavities, pneumonia, and gonorrhea, and other diseases.

*Kills fungi and yeasts that cause candidiasis, ringworm, athlete's foot, thrush, diaper rash, and other infections.

*Expels or kills tapeworms, lice, giardia, and other parasites.

*Helps prevent periodontal disease and tooth decay.

Energy

*Provides a nutritional source of quick energy.

*Boosts energy and endurance, enhancing physical and athletic performance.

Digestion and Metabolism

*Improves digestion and absorption of other nutrients including vitamins, minerals, and amino acids.

*Improves insulin secretion and utilization of blood glucose.

*Relieves stress on pancreas and enzyme systems of the body.

*Reduces symptoms associated with pancreatitis.

*Helps relieve symptoms and reduce health risks associated with diabetes.

*Reduces problems associated with malabsorption syndrome and cystic fibrosis.

*Improves calcium and magnesium absorption and supports the development of strong bones and teeth.

Helps protect against osteoporosis.

Helps relieve symptoms associated with gallbladder disease.

Relieves symptoms associated with Crohn's disease, ulcerative colitis, and stomach ulcers.

Improves digestion and bowel function. (Clients tell me that taken 20 minutes before a meal, it relieves symptoms of heartburn and GERD.)

Relieves pain and irritation caused by hemorrhoids.

Boosts the Immune System

Supports and aids immune system function.

Reduces inflammation.

Supports tissue healing and repair.

Helps protect the body from breast, colon, and other cancers.

Functions as a protective antioxidant.

Does not form harmful by-products when heated to normal cooking temperature like other vegetable oils do.

Helps to protect the body from harmful free radicals that promote premature aging and degenerative disease.

Does not deplete the body's antioxidant reserves like other oils do.

Improves utilization of essential fatty acids and protects them from oxidation.

Helps relieve symptoms associated with chronic fatigue syndrome.

Relieves symptoms associated with benign prostatic hyperplasia (prostate enlargement).

Heart Health

Is heart healthy; improves cholesterol ratio reducing risk of heart disease.

Protects arteries from injury that causes atherosclerosis and thus protects against heart disease.

Organ Support

Helps protect against kidney disease and bladder infections.

Dissolves kidney stones.

Helps prevent liver disease.

Supports thyroid function.

Reduces epileptic seizures.

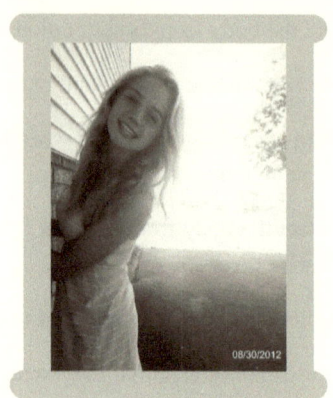

Balances Body Weight

Promotes loss of excess weight by increasing metabolic rate.

Is utilized by the body to produce energy in preference to being stored as body fat like other dietary fats.

Helps prevent obesity and overweight problems.

Is lower in calories than all other fats.

Creates Healthy Skin and Hair

Applied topically helps to form a chemical barrier on the skin to ward of infection.

Reduces symptoms associated the psoriasis, eczema, and dermatitis.

Supports the natural chemical balance of the skin.

Softens skin and helps relieve dryness and flaking.

Prevents wrinkles, sagging skin, and age spots.

Promotes healthy looking hair and complexion.

Provides protection from damaging effects of ultraviolet radiation from the sun.

Helps control dandruff.

I've also heard many anecdotal stories of coconut being used externally and internally for pets. Dogs and cats with debilitating skin rashes can be cured within days by applying coconut oil to their skin. If they lick it off, they get more benefits, not side effects as they would with cortisone creams. I have also used this on my dog when she itched one summer. I couldn't find any fleas and thought it might be dry skin. I rubbed her with Coconut Oil and found by the next day that the itching was almost gone. I noticed that she liked to lick it too so I knew she was getting the benefits of it.

What kind and how much coconut oil can you take to treat and prevent Alzheimer's and many other health conditions and treat hundreds of symptoms? The dosage used in most Alzheimer's studies is about 5 TBSP per day of extra virgin coconut oil. However, I was told that 1-3 TBSP is recommended for minor ailments and for maintenance.

How do you use coconut oil? You can substitute it in most recipes calling for oil; put it in your smoothie or protein powder drink (which is how I take it); or take it straight from the spoon.

Here's my favorite coconut recipe. Heat a Tablespoon each of coconut oil, coconut milk, cacao and a half teaspoon of honey and coat a frozen banana. You can roll it in coconut flakes and ground macadamia nuts then freeze for another 30 minutes. It makes a delicious coconut-saturated frozana!

What is the difference between coconut oil and coconut butter?

- Coconut oil is JUST the oil that is extracted from the meat.

- Coconut butter is the whole meat of the coconut pureed into a creamy butter.

- Coconut meat (by nature) is approximately 65% oil.

Before I go any further I want to share an Artisana brand of what they call Coconut Butter. I took a snippet from the Artisana site that describes their product, which is indeed different in consistency than the oil. Shoot, right now I have a jar of it in front of me on the coffee table with a spoon in it. I have been nibbling on it off and on. I can't do that with coconut oil because to me that is too oily.

Artisana Raw Coconut Butter

- Warm it up, mix it up, and spread the flavor! Freshly made from whole coconut flesh, Raw Coconut Butter is a whole food, not just oil. This delicious "cream" melts in your mouth with full coconut flavor and aroma, while giving you whole coconut nutrition: oil, dietary fiber, protein, vitamins, and minerals. No additives—only pure, unadulterated coconut.

- Artisana calls this Raw Coconut Butter a "butter" because it has more in common with nut butters than coconut oil. That's because it is made from the whole flesh of the coconut; it's also spreadable when slightly soft. Others call it coconut cream because it is so creamy when soft. Everyone, however, calls it delicious and unbelievable!

- Raw Coconut Butter is soft at above 80° F. and solid at lower temperatures. You can soften it by putting the jar inside a bowl of warm water; then stir well for a creamy, smooth texture.

- Add it to smoothies, fruit salads, sauces, salad dressings, and baked goods. Use it as a topping for ice cream, mix with cacao nibs or fruit to create your own dessert sensations, or eat it right out of the jar. Delectable!

- Raw Coconut Butter is made using a low-temperature process (below 115° F.) that preserves the vital enzymes, vitamins, and proteins. It is made from 100%

certified organic coconut, with no preservatives or other additives, in a facility that does not process any peanut, gluten, or dairy products.

- Ingredients: Organic, raw coconut

Nutiva Organic Coconut Manna (butter)

It is a whole-food product, meaning it is 100% coconut with very little processing. The difference between this and coconut oil is that coconut oil is put through a cold expresser process to get the oil out. Both are fresh-harvest coconuts that are dried, but the Manna is ground into a very fine powder right after drying. Then, they add some of their coconut oil. Manna is lower in calories than coconut oil. Nutiva Organic Coconut Manna contains 12% fiber and 9% protein, whereas coconut oil contains none.

You need to soften the product and mix thoroughly to truly appreciate the full spectrum of this amazing product. It must be softened by achieving a temperature above 76 degrees and then mixed thoroughly. If you live in a warm climate, you won't have to worry about softening. To soften:

1. Run tap water to the very hottest setting, then fill a bowl and put the Manna container in the bowl for 10-15 minutes. You may need to replace the water several times to get the butter real soft.

2. Boil water in a tea kettle and pour into a large bowl, placing the mana jar in the center. Allow it to soften.

3. If you have a food dehydrator, open the lid of the Manna container and put it in the dehydrator on 105 degrees. After 15 minutes, stir the Manna, and then put back in for another 15 minutes, then mix well before serving.

Can I substitute Coconut Oil for Coconut Butter in recipes?

The answer is not a straight yes or no. In the mainstream of things, the two are considered the same, but in the raw world having such manufacturers such as Artisana who makes a different product than coconut oil which they call coconut butter. So, for those who are not aware or don't have access to this product line, it is my belief that many people are referring to the same ingredient when they say coconut butter or coconut cream. Following me here? The Artisanan Coconut

Butter has a different flavor and texture than the coconut oils that most recipe makers are using. As a safe rule of thumb, if you are reading a recipe and they use either coconut oil or coconut butter as the ingredient terminology, I would safely assume that they are indeed using coconut oil. If you are really perplexed and want to know for sure, email or contact that recipe designer and ask them to clarify. I have used the Artisana brand of coconut butter in place of coconut oil due to what I had on hand at the time, and the recipe still came out great in the end.

Benefits of Raw Virgin Coconut Oil

Coconut oil contains absolutely no trans fats. Although many people mistakenly believe coconut oil is dangerous to health due to its saturated fat content, close to two-thirds of its saturated fat is made up of medium-chain fatty acids, which are actually health promoting and they are antimicrobial, easily digested for quick energy, and beneficial to the immune system.

The popular misconceptions about coconut oil can be traced to some decades-old flawed studies, some of which used hydrogenated (chemically altered, unnatural) coconut oils, and to misleading advertising campaigns generated by the edible oil industry. The industry instead promoted polyunsaturated fats (such as canola, soybean, safflower. and corn), which easily go rancid when exposed to oxygen and produce harmful free radicals in our bodies. Coconut oil was falsely accused of leading to coronary heart disease, a myth that has been refuted by a large body of research showing that consumption of natural coconut oil is beneficial to health, including cardiovascular health.

Traditional wisdom also supports the regular use of coconut oil. It has been used as a traditional food by the Polynesians since ancient times, and they have among the lowest rates of heart disease in the world.

Some of the health benefits of consuming coconut oil include:

- Promotes weight loss and helps maintain healthy body weight

- Reduces the risk of heart disease

- Supports thyroid function

- Increases metabolism and energy

- Prevents bacterial, viral, and fungal infections

- Helps control diabetes and chronic fatigue

- Improves digestive disorders such as Crohn's disease and IBS

- Protects against alcohol damage to the liver

- Rejuvenates skin and prevents wrinkles

Lauric acid, known for its antiviral, antibacterial, and antiprotozoal functions, makes up about 50% of the fatty acid in coconut fat. In the body, it is converted to monolaurin, a powerful monoglyceride that destroys lipid-coated viruses (such as HIV, herpes, cytomegalovirus, and influenza) as well as pathogenic bacteria including helicobacter pylori and listeria monocytogenes.

Coconut oil can vary widely in both quality and effectiveness. Most commercial coconut oils are refined, bleached, and deodorized, and many are made from "copra," or dried coconut meat. Some are even hydrogenated. Others that are called "cold-pressed" still are fermented or heated to remove water, and in the process they lose the natural vitamin E and tocopherols needed for stability and protection against rancidity.

So look for coconut oil that is virgin, cold-pressed, vitamin E rich, "biologically pure" coconut oil that is identical to unextracted oil from coconuts. To make virgin coconut oil, fresh coconut meat is grated and expeller-pressed to produce coconut milk, which is then centrifuged to separate it into solid components, oil, and water with no heating, refining, bleaching, or deodorizing.

This book is the first book in a series of books that will tell you all about keeping healthy and at a reasonable cost. If you take care of your body by eating right and taking the right Vitamins and Herbs you will feel the difference it will make. My life has changed because I took time to start watching the food I ate and taking Vitamins. Now I wouldn't be without Coconut Oil as it is a big part of my daily routine with my hair and complexion.

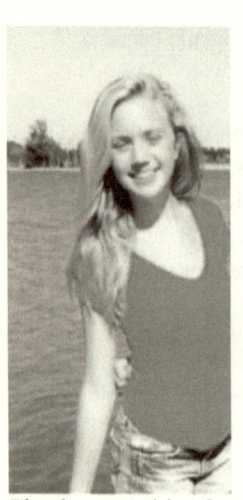

My next book in this Series will be on Make Up and how we can benefit by making our own.

We will learn of the different lotions and what is best for your body.

Also, we will show you how to make your own lotions, lipsticks, and perfume oils.

Have a great day.

Thank you Ashley for the beautiful pictures..

All proceeds from this book will go to help

Hannah House

MPO Box 2813,

Niagara Falls, New York

14302

http://hannahhouse2002.org

hannahhouse2002@gmail.com

Division of Lighthouse International Ministries.